WORLD HEALTH STATISTICS
2007

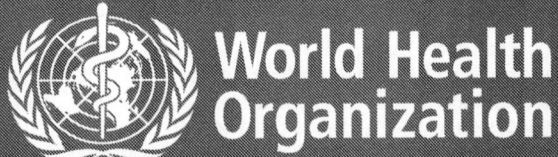

WHO Library Cataloguing-in-Publication Data

World health statistics 2007.

1.Health status indicators. 2.World health. 3.Health services - statistics. 4.Mortality. 5.Life expectancy. 6.Demography. 7.Statistics. I.World Health Organization.

ISBN 978 92 4 156340 6 (NLM classification: WA 900.1)
ISBN 978 92 4 068211 5 (electronic version)

© **World Health Organization 2007**

All rights reserved. Publications of the World Health Organization can be obtained from WHO Press, World Health Organization, 20 Avenue Appia, 1211 Geneva 27, Switzerland (tel.: +41 22 791 3264; fax: +41 22 791 4857; e-mail: bookorders@who.int). Requests for permission to reproduce or translate WHO publications – whether for sale or for noncommercial distribution – should be addressed to WHO Press, at the above address (fax: +41 22 791 4806; e-mail: permissions@who.int).

The designations employed and the presentation of the material in this publication do not imply the expression of any opinion whatsoever on the part of the World Health Organization concerning the legal status of any country, territory, city or area or of its authorities, or concerning the delimitation of its frontiers or boundaries. Dotted lines on maps represent approximate border lines for which there may not yet be full agreement.

The mention of specific companies or of certain manufacturers' products does not imply that they are endorsed or recommended by the World Health Organization in preference to others of a similar nature that are not mentioned. Errors and omissions excepted, the names of proprietary products are distinguished by initial capital letters.

All reasonable precautions have been taken by the World Health Organization to verify the information contained in this publication. However, the published material is being distributed without warranty of any kind, either expressed or implied. The responsibility for the interpretation and use of the material lies with the reader. In no event shall the World Health Organization be liable for damages arising from its use.

This publication was produced by the Department of Measurement and Health Information Systems of the Information, Evidence and Research Cluster, under the overall direction of Ties Boerma and Kenji Shibuya, in collaboration with WHO technical programmes and regional offices, and assisted by Zoe Brillantes, Maria Guraiib, Mie Inoue, Yohannes Kinfu and Doris Ma Fat.

Valuable inputs to the statistical highlights in Part 1 were received from Monika Bloessner, Ties Boerma, Somnath Chatterji, Mercedes de Onis, Christopher Dye, Christopher Fitzpatrick, Charu Garg, Mehran Hosseini, Ahmadreza Hosseinpoor, Mie Inoue, Yohannes Kinfu, Doris Ma Fat, Colin Mathers, Ritu Sadana, Kenji Shibuya, Tessa Tan-Torres and Catherine Watt. Maps were produced by the Public Health Mapping and Geographic Information Systems team, Communicable Disease and Surveillance.

Contributors to the statistical tables in Part 2 were: Michel Beusenberg, Monika Bloessner, Cynthia Boschi Pinto, Claire Chauvin, Mercedes de Onis, Christopher Dye, Christopher Fitzpatrick, Marta Gacic Dobo, Charu Garg, Chika Hayashi, Mehran Hosseini, Ahmadreza Hosseinpoor, Chandika Indikadahena, Mie Inoue, Yohannes Kinfu, Teena Kunjumen, Doris Ma Fat, Colin Mathers, Chizuru Nishida, Vladimir Pozniak, Eva Rehfuess, Dag Rekve, Leanne Riley, Lale Say, Kenji Shibuya, Jonathan Siekmann, Jacqueline Sims, Yves Souteyrand, Tessa Tan-Torres, Jeanette Vega, Catherine Watt, and many staff in WHO country offices, governmental departments and agencies and international institutions. Additional help and advice were kindly provided by regional offices and members of their staff, including Yok-Ching Chong, Anton Fric, Remigijus Prochorskas, Saher Shuqaidef, William Soumbey-Alley and Fernando Zacarias.

The publication was edited by Miriam Pinchuk. Editorial and production support was provided by the Department of Knowledge Management and Sharing, including Caroline Allsopp, Ian Coltart, Laragh Gollogly, Maryvonne Grisetti, Sophie Guetaneh Aguettant, Hooman Momen, and Catherine Roch. The web site version and other electronic media were provided by the Digital Publishing Solution, Ltd. Proofreading was by Melanie Lauckner. We also thank Susan Piccolo and Petra Schuster for their administrative support.

Printed in France

Table of Contents

Introduction	**7**

Part 1. Ten statistical highlights in global public health	**9**
1. Monitoring progress: appropriate use of health statistics	10
2. People living with HIV: better data, better estimates	11
3. Future health: projected deaths for selected causes to 2030	12
4. Child undernutrition: where are we now?	13
5. Levels and causes of death: filling data gaps	14
6. Tobacco use and poverty: high prevalence among the world's poorest	15
7. Mental illness: depression worsens the health of people with chronic illness	16
8. Inequalities in health: understanding their determinants	17
9. Tuberculosis control: towards goals and targets	18
10. Health expenditure: meeting needs?	19
References	20

Part 2. World health statistics	**21**
Health status: mortality	**22**

Life expectancy at birth (years)
Healthy life expectancy (HALE) at birth (years)
Probability of dying aged 15–60 years per 1 000 population (adult mortality rate)
Probability of dying aged < 5 years per 1 000 live births (under-5 mortality rate)
Infant mortality rate (per 1 000 live births)
Neonatal mortality rate (per 1 000 live births)
Maternal mortality ratio (per 100 000 live births)
Deaths due to HIV/AIDS (per 100 000 population per year)
Deaths due to tuberculosis among HIV-negative people (per 100 000 population per year)
Deaths due to tuberculosis among HIV-positive people (per 100 000 population per year)
Age-standardized mortality rate by cause (per 100 000 population)
Distribution of years of life lost by broader causes (%)
Distribution of causes of death among children aged < 5 years (%)

Health status: morbidity	**32**

HIV prevalence among adults aged ≥ 15 years (per 100 000 population)
Prevalence of tuberculosis (per 100 000 population)
Incidence of tuberculosis (per 100 000 population per year)
Number of confirmed cases of poliomyelitis

Table of Contents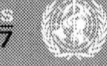

Health service coverage   36

Immunization coverage among 1-year-olds with one dose of measles (%)
Immunization coverage among 1-year-olds with three doses of diphtheria, tetanus toxoid and pertussis (DTP3) (%)
Immunization coverage among 1-year-olds with three doses of Hepatitis B (HepB3) (%)
Antenatal care coverage (%)
Births attended by skilled health personnel (%)
Contraceptive prevalence rate (%)
Children aged < 5 years sleeping under insecticide-treated bednets (%)
Antiretroviral therapy coverage among people with advanced HIV infections (%)
HIV-infected pregnant women who received antiretrovirals for PMTCT (%)
Tuberculosis detection rate under DOTS (%)
Tuberculosis treatment success under DOTS (%)
Children aged < 5 years with ARI symptoms taken to facility (%)
Children aged < 5 years with diarrhoea receiving ORT (%)
Children aged < 5 years with fever who received treatment with any antimalarial (%)
Children 6–59 months who received vitamin A supplementation (%)
Births by Caesarean section (%)

Risk factors   46

Children aged < 5 years stunted for age (%)
Children aged < 5 years underweight for age (%)
Children aged < 5 years overweight for age (%)
Low-birthweight newborns (%)
Adults aged ≥ 15 years who are obese (%)
Access to improved drinking water sources (%)
Access to improved sanitation (%)
Population using solid fuels (%)
Prevalence of current tobacco use in adolescents (13–15 years) (%)
Prevalence of current tobacco use among adults (≥ 15 years) (%)
Per capita recorded alcohol consumption (litres of pure alcohol) among adults (≥ 15 years)
Prevalence of condom use by young people (15–24 years) at higher risk sex (%)

Health systems   56

Human resources for health   56
   Physicians; Nurses; Midwives; Dentists; Pharmacists; Public and environmental health workers; Community health workers; Laboratory health workers; Other health workers; Health management and support workers

Table of Contents

Health expenditure ratios — 64
  Total expenditure on health as % of gross domestic product
  General government expenditure on health as % of total expenditure on health
  Private expenditure on health as % of total expenditure on health
  General government expenditure on health as % of total government expenditure
  External resources for health as % of total expenditure on health
  Social security expenditure on health as % of general government expenditure on health
  Out-of-pocket expenditure as % of private expenditure on health
  Private prepaid plans as % of private expenditure on health
Health expenditure aggregates
  Per capita total expenditure on health at average exchange rate (US$) — 65
  Per capita total expenditure on health at international dollar rate
  Per capita government expenditure on health at average exchange rate (US$)
  Per capita government expenditure on health at international dollar rate
Coverage of vital registration of deaths (%) — 65
Hospital beds (per 10 000 population) — 65

Inequities in health — 74

Probability of dying aged < 5 years per 1 000 live births (under-5 mortality rate)
by place of residence; by wealth quintile; by educational level of mother
Children aged < 5 years stunted for age (%)
by place of residence; by wealth quintile; by educational level of mother
Births attended by skilled health personnel (%)
by place of residence; by wealth quintile; by educational level of mother
Measles immunization coverage among 1-year-olds
by place of residence; by wealth quintile; by educational level of mother

Demographic and socioeconomic statistics — 78

Population (thousands)
Annual population growth rate (%)
Population in urban areas (%)
Total fertility rate (per woman)
Adolescent fertility rate (%)
Adult literacy rate (%)
Net primary school enrolment ratio (%)
Gross national income per capita (international$)
Population living below the poverty line (% living on < US$1 per day)

Introduction

World health statistics 2007 presents the most recent health statistics for WHO's 193 Member States. This third edition includes a section with 10 highlights of global health statistics for the past year as well as an expanded set of 50 health statistics.

World health statistics 2007 has been collated from publications and databases produced by WHO's technical programmes and regional offices. The core set of indicators was selected on the basis of their relevance to global health, the availability and quality of the data, and the accuracy and comparability of estimates. The statistics for the indicators are derived from an interactive process of data collection, compilation, quality assessment and estimation occurring among WHO's technical programmes and its Member States. During this process, WHO strives to maximize the accessibility, accuracy, comparability and transparency of health statistics.[1]

In addition to national statistics, this publication presents statistics on the distribution of selected health outcomes and interventions within countries, disaggregated by gender, age, urban versus rural setting, wealth, and educational level. Such statistics are primarily derived from analyses of household surveys and are available only for a limited number of countries. We envisage that the number of countries reporting disaggregated data will increase during the next few years.

The core indicators do not aim to capture all relevant aspects of health but to provide a comprehensive summary of the current status of a population's health and the health system at country level. These indicators include: mortality outcomes, morbidity outcomes, risk factors, coverage of selected health interventions, health systems, inequalities in health, and demographic and socioeconomic statistics.

All statistics have been cleared as WHO's official figures in consultation with Member States unless otherwise stated. WHO's estimates use data from publicly accessible databases, peer-reviewed methods of estimation, and consultation with experts around the world. The estimates published here should, however, still be regarded as best estimates made by WHO rather than the official view of Member States.

As the demand for timely, reliable and comparable information on key health statistics continues to increase, users need to be well informed about the definitions used and the quality and limitations of health statistics. More detailed information, including a compendium of statistics and an online version of this publication, is available from WHO's Statistical Information System (http://www.who.int/statistics). The web site also includes information on how each statistic is derived.

The online version of *World health statistics 2007* will be updated regularly, and it includes the most recent estimates and time-series of relevant health statistics. The online version also provides, whenever possible, metadata describing the sources of data, estimation methods and quality of estimates. It is hoped that careful scrutiny and use of the statistics presented in this report will lead to progressively better measurement of relevant indicators of population health and health systems.

---

1. To meet these objectives, WHO has initiated the organization-wide Programme on Health Statistics. For more information, see http://www.who.int/healthinfo/statistics/programme/en/index.html.

Part 1
Ten statistical highlights in global public health

1. Monitoring progress: appropriate use of health statistics

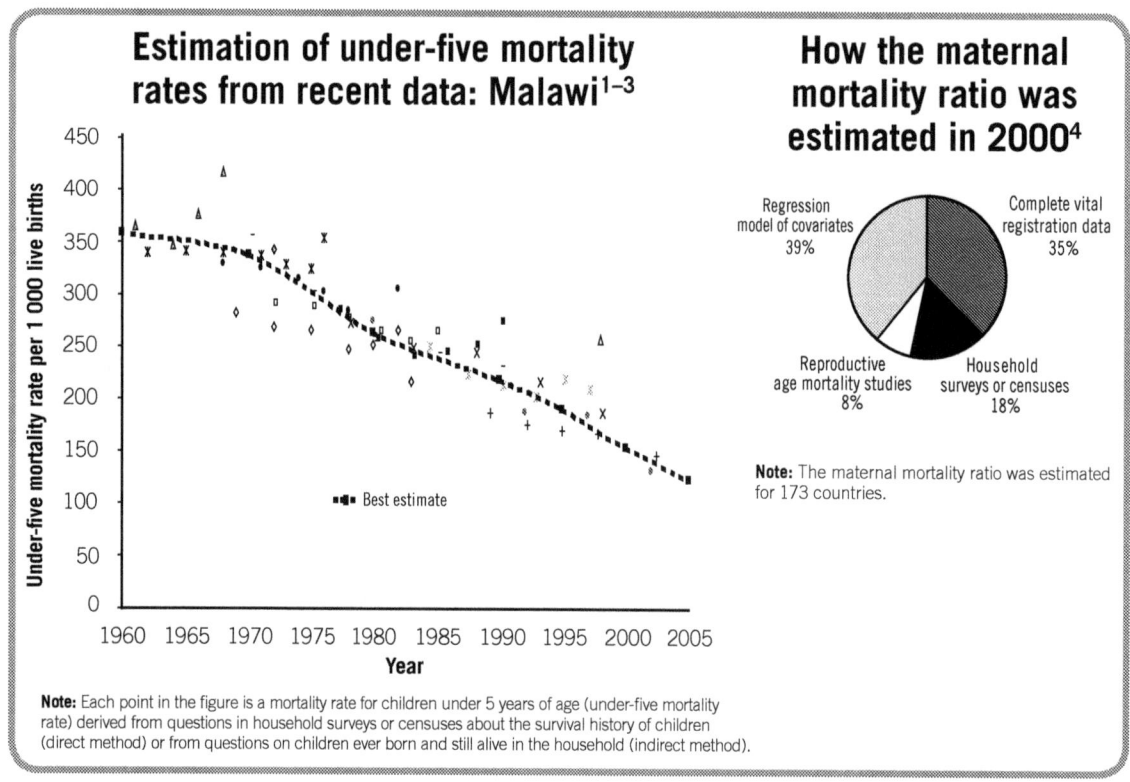

Estimation of under-five mortality rates from recent data: Malawi[1–3]

How the maternal mortality ratio was estimated in 2000[4]

Note: The maternal mortality ratio was estimated for 173 countries.

Note: Each point in the figure is a mortality rate for children under 5 years of age (under-five mortality rate) derived from questions in household surveys or censuses about the survival history of children (direct method) or from questions on children ever born and still alive in the household (indirect method).

The ability to monitor progress towards the Millennium Development Goals (MDGs) depends primarily on data availability. There is a stark contrast between the data available about the under-five mortality rate, the indicator for MDG 4, and the maternal mortality ratio, against which MDG 5 is monitored.

Under-five mortality rates are derived from vital registration systems, censuses and household surveys.[1] In most countries, there are data points available over time, and these are analysed to obtain the best current estimate. Uncertainty occurs when there is a need to project estimates forward to the current year since the most recent data generally refer to a few years earlier. Measuring the maternal mortality ratio has been a greater challenge because, compared with deaths among children, maternal deaths are rare events. In countries without a complete death registration system and medical certification, large-scale household surveys or censuses using verbal autopsy techniques provide estimates of the ratio, since facility-based statistics are inherently biased. Even then, much uncertainty remains. As a consequence, the global estimate of the maternal mortality ratio is published only once every five years, and in 2000, 40% of countries' estimates were based on figures predicted by regression.[4] The ability to reliably assess trends in maternal mortality is limited.

For monitoring, it is important to distinguish between corrected and predicted statistics.[5,6] Corrected statistics use adjustments made for known biases and, if needed, are based on a systematic reconciliation of data from multiple sources using established, transparent methods. Predicted statistics use a set of assumptions about the association between other factors and the quantity of interest, such as maternal mortality, to fill gaps in the data over time (projecting into the present or future) or space (from one population with data to another with limited or no data). Predicted statistics are not suitable for monitoring progress. Unfortunately, the MDG monitoring process relies heavily on predicted statistics.[5] This mismatch was created partly by the demand for more timely statistics and partly by the lack of data and good measurement strategies for certain statistics. It is crucial for the international community to invest in data collection and use indicators that are valid, reliable and comparable; the international community must also have well-defined measurement strategies for monitoring progress and evaluating health programmes.[7]

2. People living with HIV: better data, better estimates

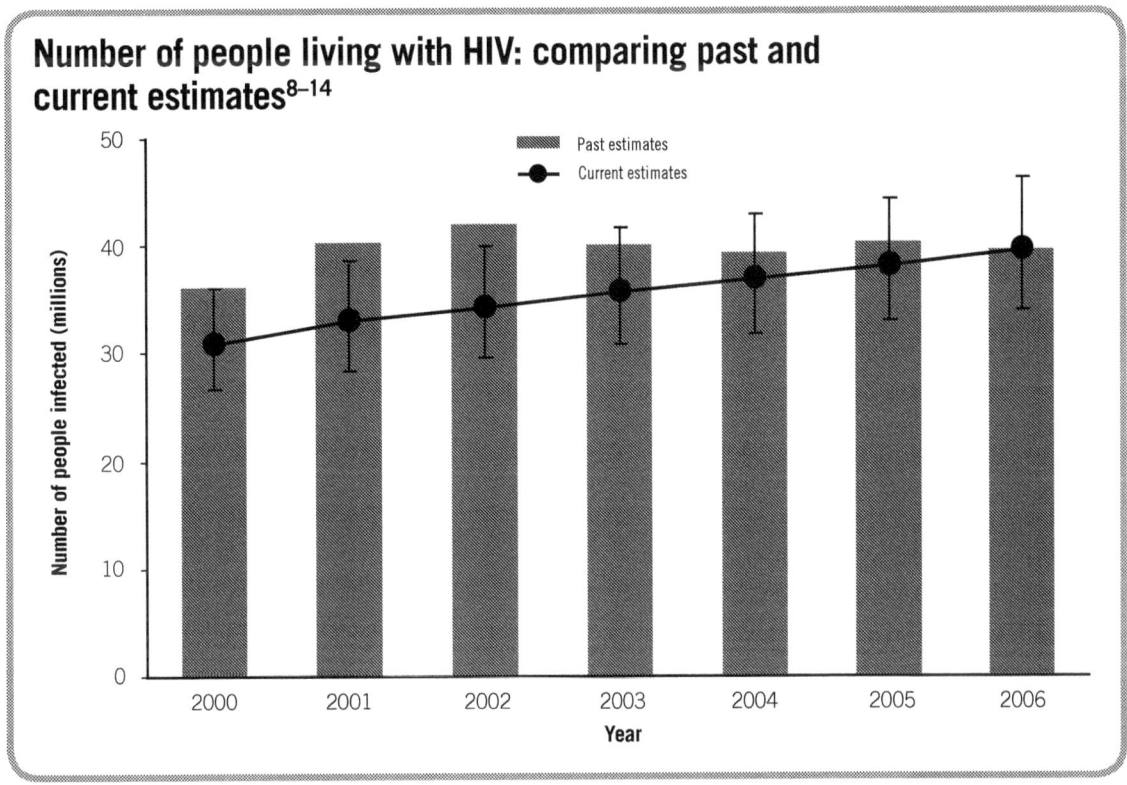

Number of people living with HIV: comparing past and current estimates[8-14]

The exact number of people living with HIV is unknown despite the fact that HIV infection can easily be diagnosed by a widely used antibody test. Achieving 100% certainty about the number of people living with HIV globally would require testing every person in the world for HIV every year. Nonetheless, we can estimate the number by using data from different sources, such as surveillance of pregnant women attending antenatal clinics, household surveys with HIV testing and sentinel surveillance among populations at higher risk of HIV infection.

UNAIDS and WHO, in close consultation with countries, employ a standardized method for obtaining estimates of HIV prevalence among men and women. An increasing number of countries have adopted these methods to develop their own national estimates. But an estimate is only as good as the data. As more complete data become available, past estimates may need to be adjusted. This is the case for the AIDS epidemic. The bars in the figure estimate the number of people infected with HIV at the time of publication of each annual *AIDS epidemic update* since 2000.[8-14] The line shows the best estimates for each year that were made in 2006 in the most recent update: this reveals not only that the size of the epidemic had been overestimated previously but also that it is still growing. The ranges around the estimates reflect the degree of uncertainty about global HIV estimates.

Improvements in recent estimates are the result of revisions made using better data. These revisions used data from national population-based surveys and benefited from improvements in the quality and coverage of sentinel surveillance systems in many countries.

The latest estimates cannot be compared directly with estimates published previously. It would be incorrect to derive a trend by comparing the bars. The 2006 estimates for this year and past years (indicated by the line) are more accurate than those produced in previous years since they are based on improved methods and used more data than earlier estimates. The need to exercise caution is not unusual when comparing global estimates of disease over time.

3. Future health: projected deaths for selected causes to 2030

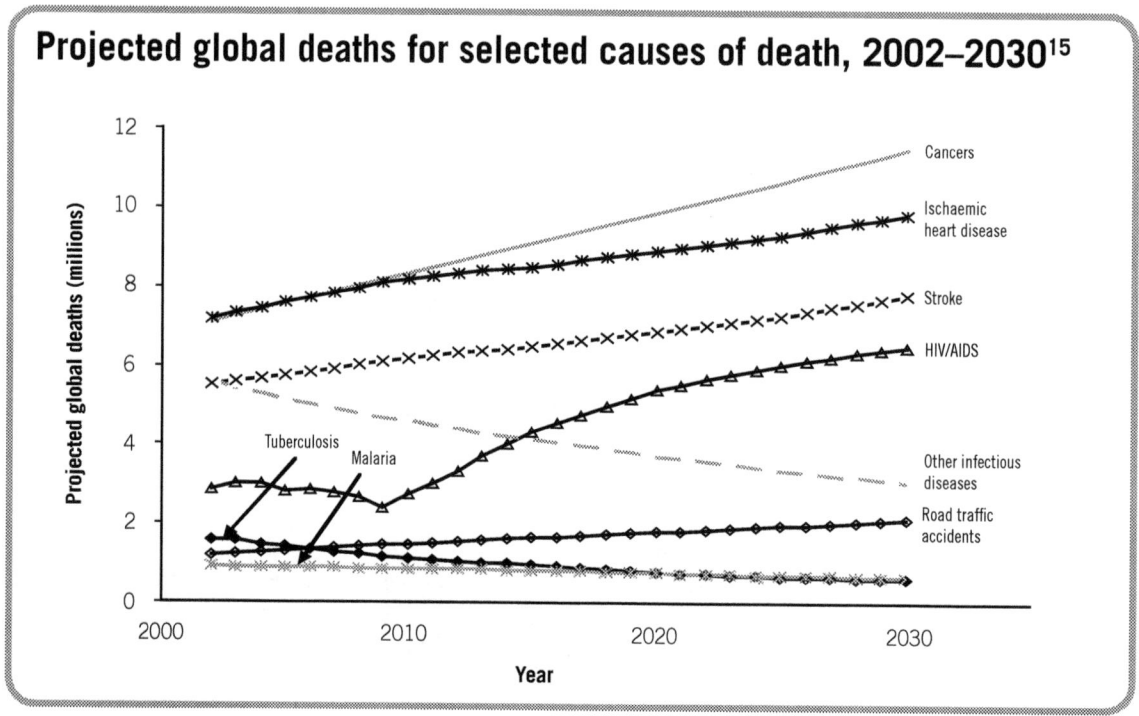

Projected global deaths for selected causes of death, 2002–2030[15]

Predicted statistics have an important and useful role in helping to inform planning and strategic decision-making, and in prioritizing research and development issues. According to projections carried out by WHO and published in early 2006,[15] the world will experience a substantial shift in the distribution of deaths from younger age groups to older age groups, and from communicable diseases to noncommunicable diseases during the next 25 years. Large declines in mortality are projected to occur between 2002 and 2030 for all of the principal communicable, maternal, perinatal and nutritional causes, with the exception of HIV/AIDS. Global deaths from HIV/AIDS are projected to rise from 2.8 million in 2002 to 6.5 million in 2030 under a baseline scenario that assumes antiretroviral drug coverage reaches 80% by 2012.

Although age-specific death rates for most noncommunicable diseases are projected to decline, the ageing of the global population will result in significant increases in the total number of deaths caused by most noncommunicable diseases over the next 30 years. Overall, noncommunicable conditions will account for almost 70% of all deaths in 2030 under the baseline scenario. The projected 40% increase in global deaths resulting from injury between 2002 and 2030 is predominantly due to the increasing number of deaths from road traffic accidents.

The four leading causes of death globally in 2030 are projected to be ischaemic heart disease, cerebrovascular disease (stroke), HIV/AIDS and chronic obstructive pulmonary disease. The total number of tobacco-attributable deaths is projected to rise from 5.4 million in 2005 to 6.4 million in 2015 and to 8.3 million in 2030. Tobacco is projected to kill 50% more people in 2015 than HIV/AIDS and to be responsible for 10% of all deaths.

4. Child undernutrition: where are we now?

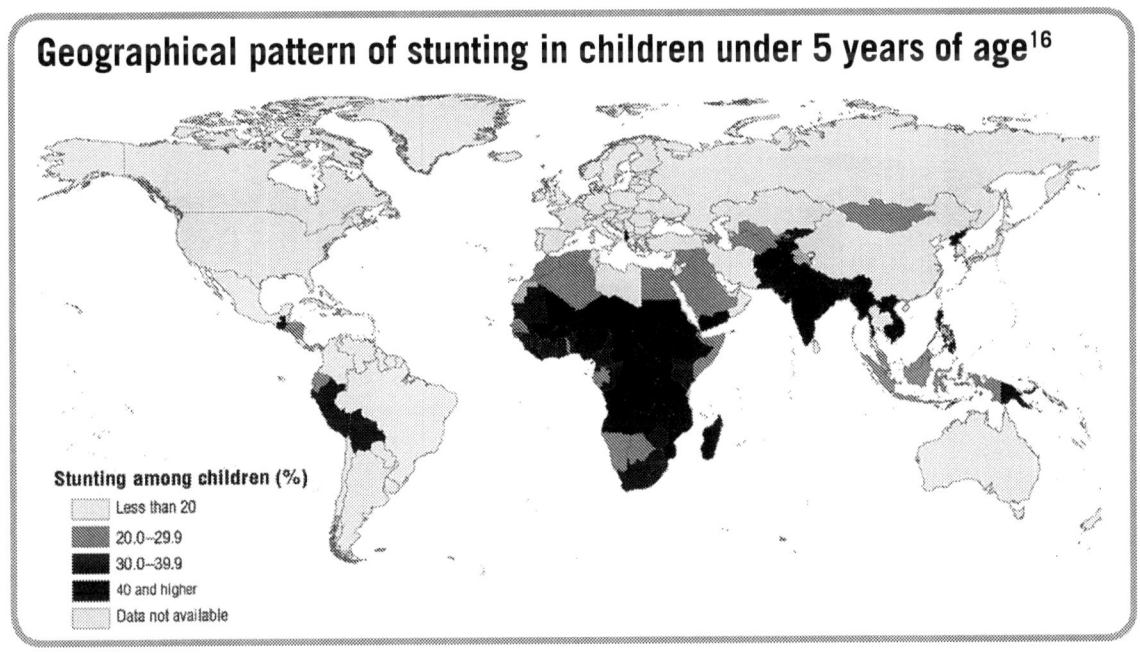

Geographical pattern of stunting in children under 5 years of age[16]

Stunting among children (%)
- Less than 20
- 20.0–29.9
- 30.0–39.9
- 40 and higher
- Data not available

The release of WHO's new Child Growth Standards (http://www.who.int/childgrowth/en) has an impact on estimates of undernutrition among children. Global, regional and country estimates have been recalculated using the new standards, which include data from 388 national surveys in 139 countries.[16]

In 2005, in all developing countries 32% of children under 5 years of age (178 million children) were estimated to be stunted (that is, their height fell –2 standard deviations below the median height-for-age of the reference population). In that year, more than 40% of stunting was found in the WHO regions of Africa and South-East Asia, around 25% in the Eastern Mediterranean Region and 10–15% in the regions of the Americas and the Western Pacific. Of the 39 countries with a prevalence of stunting of 40% and higher, 22 are in the African Region, 7 in South-East Asia, 4 in the Eastern Mediterranean, 4 in the Western Pacific, and 1 each in Europe and in the Americas. Of the 35 countries with a stunting prevalence lower than 20%, 13 are in the Region of the Americas, 11 in Europe, 6 in the Eastern Mediterranean, 3 in the Western Pacific and 2 in South-East Asia.

Wasting (defined as being –2 standard deviations below the median of weight-for-height) is a sign of acute malnutrition and is a strong predictor of mortality among children. The global estimate of wasting occurring among children under 5 years of age based on WHO's new standards is 10% (or 55 million). The highest number of affected children – 29 million – is estimated to live in south–central Asia. The same regional pattern is found for severe wasting (defined as being –3 standard deviations below the median), with an estimated total prevalence of 4% – or 19 million – children affected. Many of these children are likely to die before reaching the age of 5 years. In general, compared with estimates based on the previous international reference, stunting rates are higher for all age groups when the new WHO standards are used. Additionally, the prevalences of wasting and severe wasting are higher during the first half of infancy with the new WHO standards; and thereafter severe wasting rates continue to be 1.5 to 2.5 times higher than those of the previous reference.

5. Levels and causes of death: filling data gaps

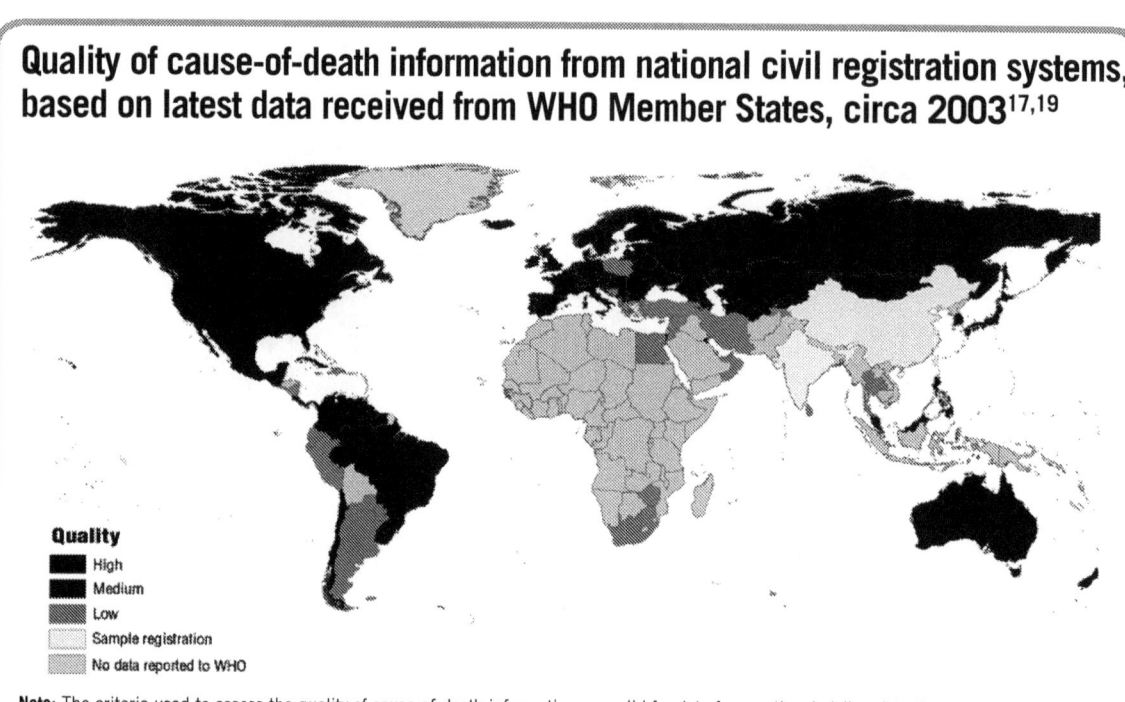

Quality of cause-of-death information from national civil registration systems, based on latest data received from WHO Member States, circa 2003[17,19]

Note: The criteria used to assess the quality of cause-of-death information are valid for data from national civil registration systems. Therefore, they do not apply to China and India since they report data from sample registration systems, which cover < 10% of their populations.

Accurate and timely data on deaths and causes of death with medical certification are essential. WHO collects information on causes of death from its Member States annually. However, for more than a fourth of the world's population – largely located in Africa, South-East Asia and the Middle East – there are no recent data available to WHO, and these are the areas where much of the burden of disease falls. Altogether, 115 Member States have some form of death registration known to WHO; this includes China and India, which also have sample vital registration systems.

There are delays in compiling, analysing and reporting these statistics: by 2007 WHO had received reports for 2004 or 2005 for 64 (56%) countries. An assessment of the quality of cause-of-death information by WHO suggested that ideal systems operate in only 29 of 115 countries that report such statistics to WHO; these systems represent less than 13% of the world's population.[17] In the remaining countries mortality statistics suffer from one or more of the following problems: incomplete registration of births and deaths, lay reporting of the cause of death, poor coverage and incorrect reporting of ages.

The ultimate goals should be to establish complete vital registration with medical certification of deaths in all countries. National governments, with the support of international organizations, need to continue to make efforts to improve the coverage and quality of vital registration systems.

At the same time, complementary approaches to complete vital registration are needed to respond to the demand for timely information and to assess the performance of the systems themselves. WHO, in collaboration with its partners, is stepping up efforts to improve the quality of data that underlies its overall estimates of mortality by age, sex and cause.[18] Such efforts include making better use of household surveys and censuses, implementing standardized verbal autopsy instruments, and using data from partial vital registration and sources other than vital registration.

6. Tobacco use and poverty: high prevalence among the world's poorest

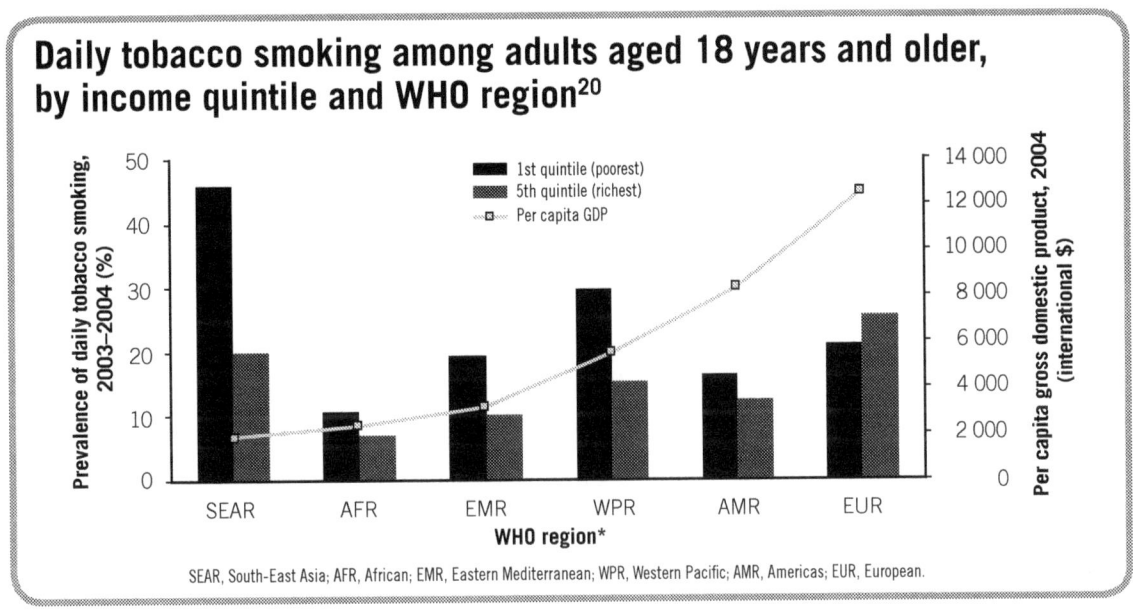

Daily tobacco smoking among adults aged 18 years and older, by income quintile and WHO region[20]

SEAR, South-East Asia; AFR, African; EMR, Eastern Mediterranean; WPR, Western Pacific; AMR, Americas; EUR, European.

Health inequalities refer to differences in health status or in the distribution of health determinants between different populations. The burden of disease attributable to tobacco use weighs increasingly heavily on populations in developing economies. According to the latest estimates, more than 80% of the 8.3 million deaths attributed to tobacco and projected to the year 2030 will occur in low-income and middle-income countries.[15]

Data on the prevalence of smoking among adults in developing countries are limited. WHO's World Health Survey provides a valuable insight into the comparative prevalence among adults aged 18 and older.[20] The results of the 2003–2004 survey indicate that daily tobacco smoking is most prevalent among the lowest-income households in developing economies – that is, among the poorest of the poor. Indeed, prevalence is highest among the poor in all WHO regions except the European Region. The difference in prevalence between the poor and the (relatively) rich is greatest among the group of South-East Asian countries surveyed, where average per capita income is lowest.

The combination of a higher prevalence of tobacco use and more limited access to health resources results in severe health inequalities, and is likely to perpetuate the vicious circle of illness and poverty. Inequalities between and within countries in terms of the risk of infectious diseases now have been extended to inequalities in risk factors for noncommunicable diseases; this has implications for health systems at all levels.

---

* Surveyed countries in each region include: African Region (AFR): Burkina Faso, Chad, Comoros, Congo, Côte d'Ivoire, Ethiopia, Ghana, Kenya, Malawi, Mali, Mauritania, Mauritius, Namibia, Senegal, South Africa, Swaziland, Zambia, Zimbabwe; Region of the Americas (AMR): Brazil, Dominican Republic, Ecuador, Guatemala, Mexico, Paraguay, Uruguay; Eastern Mediterranean Region (EMR): Morocco, Pakistan, Tunisia, United Arab Emirates; European Region (EUR): Bosnia and Herzegovina, Croatia, Czech Republic, Estonia, Georgia, Hungary, Kazakhstan, Latvia, Russian Federation, Slovakia, Slovenia, Spain, Ukraine; South-East Asia Region (SEAR): Bangladesh, India, Sri Lanka, Myanmar, Nepal; Western Pacific Region (WPR): China, Laos, Malaysia, Philippines, Viet Nam.

7. Mental illness: depression worsens the health of people with chronic illness

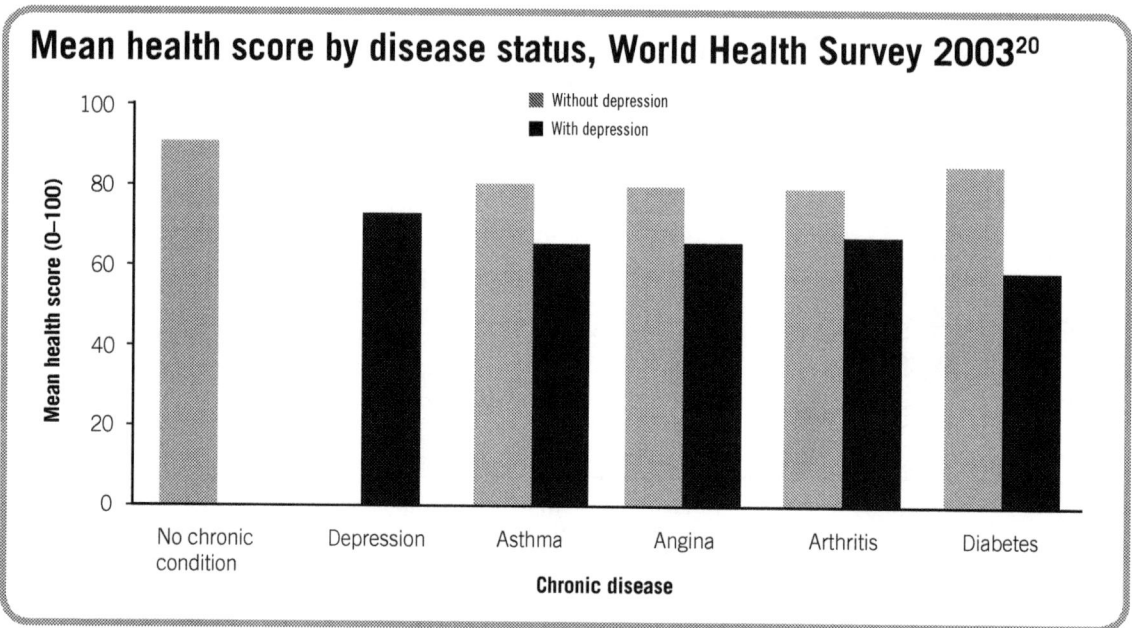

Mean health score by disease status, World Health Survey 2003[20]

Depression is an important global public health problem due to both its relatively high lifetime prevalence and the significant disability that it causes. In 2002, depression accounted for 4.5% of the worldwide total burden of disease (in terms of disability-adjusted life years). It is also responsible for the greatest proportion of burden attributable to non-fatal health outcomes, accounting for almost 12% of total years lived with disability worldwide.[21] Without treatment, depression has the tendency to assume a chronic course, to recur, and to be associated with increasing disability over time.

WHO's World Health Survey collected data on health and health-related outcomes and their determinants in samples of adults aged 18 years and older.[20] The prevalence of depression was estimated using criteria in the *International statistical classification of diseases and related health problems, tenth revision* (ICD-10). The prevalences of four chronic physical diseases – angina, arthritis, asthma and diabetes – were also estimated. The figure shows the mean health score – where 0 is the worst level of health and 100 is the best level of health – for each disease with and without accompanying depression. Individuals without depression and without other conditions had a mean health score of 90. Respondents with only one of the chronic diseases had mean health scores of around 80. Respondents with depression but without chronic disease had the lowest mean health score (73). Respondents with depression and another chronic condition had much lower mean health scores when compared with respondents who had only a chronic condition. These patterns were consistent after adjusting for sociodemographic variables.

This analysis does not tell us whether people are more depressed because they have a coexisting chronic condition. The timely diagnosis and treatment of depressive disorders are essential irrespective of causality. In many primary care settings when patients present with multiple disorders that include depression, the depression often remains undiagnosed, and even if it is diagnosed, treatment usually focuses on the other chronic diseases. Depression can be treated in primary care or community settings using locally available and cost-effective interventions.

8. Inequalities in health: understanding their determinants

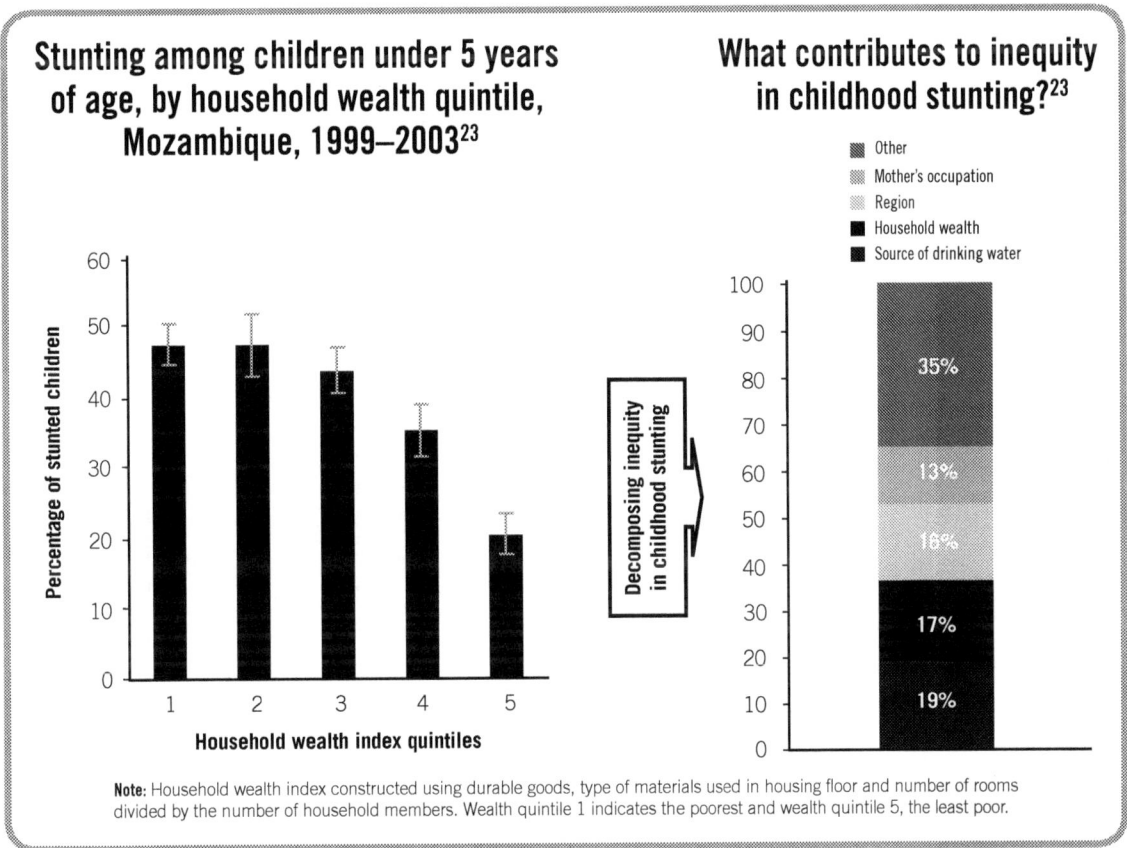

Stunting among children under 5 years of age, by household wealth quintile, Mozambique, 1999–2003[23]

What contributes to inequity in childhood stunting?[23]

Note: Household wealth index constructed using durable goods, type of materials used in housing floor and number of rooms divided by the number of household members. Wealth quintile 1 indicates the poorest and wealth quintile 5, the least poor.

Measuring socioeconomic inequalities in a population's health is important because national averages often mask differences within and across subgroups. For policy purposes it is especially relevant to understand why unfair and avoidable inequalities (or inequities) exist and what actions may be taken to improve equity. Decomposition analysis is one approach used to quantify the contribution made by different factors to inequities in health; it takes into account the socioeconomic distribution of determinants of health and health indicators.[22] Such analysis can serve as one input to aid in the development of evidence-based policies, relevant to a particular context or country, to reduce inequities.

For example, decomposition analysis using data from the 2003 Demographic and Health Survey in Mozambique shows that the four biggest contributors to poor growth in children (defined as height-for-age falling 2 standard deviations below the median of the reference population) stratified by household wealth are: source of drinking water (19%), household wealth itself (17%), geographical differences (16%) and mother's occupation (13%).[23] An additional 10 factors identified in the survey together contribute 35%. Using this technique to uncover inequities reveals that strategies to address contributing factors are likely to require collaborative and intersectoral actions that are not limited to health authorities or the health system.

Describing health inequities and understanding their determinants require process and outcome data that can be disaggregated by different socioeconomic or demographic characteristics, as well as the ability to link data from different sectors in a country. WHO is contributing to these efforts by setting norms and standards, and providing technical assistance to Member States.

9. Tuberculosis control: towards goals and targets

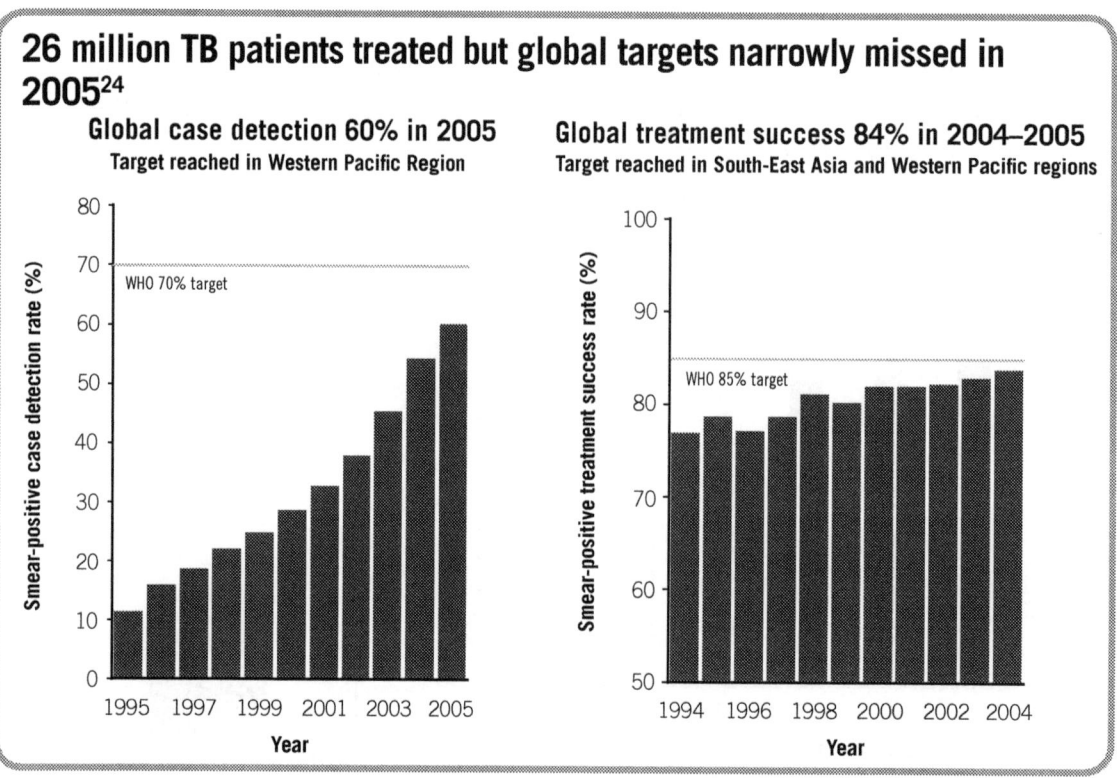

26 million TB patients treated but global targets narrowly missed in 2005[24]

Global case detection 60% in 2005
Target reached in Western Pacific Region

Global treatment success 84% in 2004–2005
Target reached in South-East Asia and Western Pacific regions

There were an estimated 8.8 million new tuberculosis (TB) cases in 2005, including 7.4 million in Asia and sub-Saharan Africa. A total of 1.6 million people died of TB, including 195 000 patients infected with HIV. Using surveillance data, *Global tuberculosis control: surveillance, planning, financing* draws four main conclusions about TB control programmes.[24]

First, although more than 26 million TB patients have been treated under WHO's DOTS strategy, the world's TB control programmes narrowly missed their 2005 targets for case detection (reaching 60% compared to the target of 70%) and cure (84% compared to the target of 85%). However, both targets were met in WHO's Western Pacific Region and in 26 countries including China, the Philippines and Viet Nam. Second, while the total number of patients diagnosed and treated in 2005 using DOTS approached the target, the number of patients known to be HIV positive or carrying multidrug-resistant TB (MDR-TB) were far fewer than anticipated by *The Global Plan to Stop TB 2006–2015*.[25] Therefore, major efforts are needed to step up collaborative activities between TB and HIV programmes and to manage MDR-TB and extensively drug-resistant TB. Third, the global TB epidemic appears to be on the threshold of decline. The incidence rate is now stable or falling in all WHO regions, including Africa and Europe.

These findings, if robust, mean that MDG Target 8 ("Have halted by 2015 and begun to reverse the incidence of malaria and other major diseases [including TB]") will be met before 2015. However, the total number of new cases was still rising slowly in 2005 in WHO's African, Eastern Mediterranean and South-East Asia regions. For reasons that are not fully understood, in Asian countries that report high rates of case detection and treatment success, the incidence has not been reduced as quickly as expected. This is linked to the fourth conclusion: the global burden of TB is not falling fast enough to satisfy the more demanding targets set by the Stop TB Partnership. At the current pace, 1990's prevalence and mortality rates will not be halved worldwide by 2015.

10. Health expenditure: meeting needs?

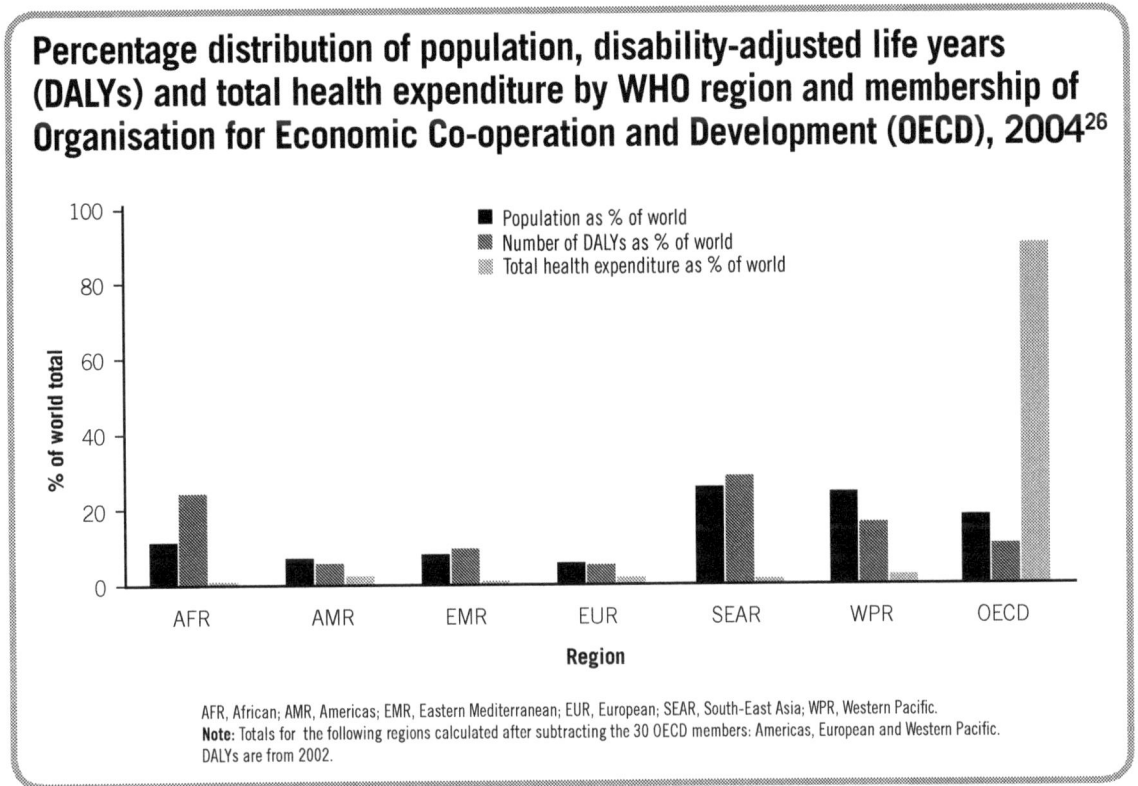

Percentage distribution of population, disability-adjusted life years (DALYs) and total health expenditure by WHO region and membership of Organisation for Economic Co-operation and Development (OECD), 2004[26]

AFR, African; AMR, Americas; EMR, Eastern Mediterranean; EUR, European; SEAR, South-East Asia; WPR, Western Pacific.
Note: Totals for the following regions calculated after subtracting the 30 OECD members: Americas, European and Western Pacific. DALYs are from 2002.

In 2004, the world spent a total of US$ 4.1 trillion on health, which is equivalent to 4.9 trillion international dollars. (International dollars are used to account for the purchasing power of different national currencies.) The geographical distribution of financial resources for health is uneven.[26] There is a 20/90 syndrome in which 30 member countries of the Organisation for Economic Co-operation and Development (OECD) make up less than 20% of the world's population but spend 90% of the world's resources on health.

OECD countries spend a larger share of their gross domestic product on health, spending on average more than 11%, compared with 4.7% for countries in WHO's African and South-East Asia regions. This translates to per capita spending of about 3080 international dollars (US$ 3170) in OECD countries compared with 102 international dollars (US$ 36) in countries in the African and South-East Asia regions, which are much poorer. Linking this spending to epidemiology, the figure shows that although poorer WHO regions, such as Africa and South-East Asia, account for the largest share of the global burden of disease (more than 50% of global disability-adjusted life years lost) and 37% of the world's population, they spend about 2% of global resources on health. The Western Pacific Region, excluding Australia, Japan, New Zealand and the Republic of Korea, accounts for 24% of the world's population (which is dominated by China), about 18% of the global burden of disease but only 2% of the world's health resources. The Region of the Americas and the European Region, excluding the OECD countries, account for about 12% of the world's population, 11% of the global burden of disease and spend slightly less than 5% of health resources.

Richer countries with smaller populations and lower disease burdens use more health resources than poorer countries with larger populations and higher disease burdens. This highlights the absolute need for additional resources for many poor countries and raises questions about the efficiency of spending on health in richer countries.

References

1. Hill K et al. Trends in child mortality in the developing world: 1990 to 1996. New York, UNICEF, 1998.
2. United Nations Children's Fund. *State of the world's children 2007.* New York, United Nations Children's Fund, 2006.
3. ORC Macro. *Demographic and health survey: Malawi 2007.* Calverton, MD, ORC Macro, 2007.
4. *Maternal mortality in 2000: estimates developed by WHO, UNICEF and UNFPA.* Geneva, World Health Organization, 2004.
5. Murray CJ. Towards good practice for health statistics: lessons from the Millennium Development Goal health indicators. *Lancet,* 2007, 369:862–873.
6. *Advisory Committee on Health Monitoring and Statistics: meeting report.* Geneva, World Health Organization, 2006 (http://www.who.int/healthinfo/statistics/healthinfoachmsreport20061214-15.pdf, accessed 4 April 2007).
7. Boerma JT, Stansfield SK. Health statistics now: are we making the right investments? *Lancet,* 2007, 369:779–786.
8. *AIDS epidemic update: December 2000.* Geneva, Joint United Nations Programme on HIV/AIDS, World Health Organization, 2000 (WHO/CDS/CSR/EDC/2000.9).
9. *AIDS epidemic update: December 2001.* Geneva, Joint United Nations Programme on HIV/AIDS, World Health Organization, 2001 (WHO/CDS/CSR/NCS/2001.2).
10. *AIDS epidemic update: December 2002.* Geneva, Joint United Nations Programme on HIV/AIDS, World Health Organization, 2002 (UNAIDS/02.58E).
11. *AIDS epidemic update: December 2003.* Geneva, Joint United Nations Programme on HIV/AIDS, World Health Organization, 2003 (UNAIDS/03.39E).
12. *AIDS epidemic update: December 2004.* Geneva, Joint United Nations Programme on HIV/AIDS, World Health Organization, 2004 (UNAIDS/04.16E).
13. *AIDS epidemic update: December 2005.* Geneva, Joint United Nations Programme on HIV/AIDS, World Health Organization, 2005 (UNAIDS/05.19E).
14. *AIDS epidemic update: December 2006.* Geneva, Joint United Nations Programme on HIV/AIDS, World Health Organization, 2006 (UNAIDS/06.29E).
15. Mathers CD, Loncar D. Projections of global mortality and burden of disease from 2002 to 2030. *PLoS Medicine* [online journal], 2006, 3(11):e442 (http://medicine.plosjournals.org/perlserv/?request=get-document&doi=10.1371/journal.pmed.0030442, accessed 4 April 2007).
16. Global database on child growth and malnutrition [online database]. Geneva, World Health Organization, 2007 (http://www.who.int/nutgrowthdb/database/en, accessed 4 April 2007).
17. Mathers CD et al. Counting the dead and what they died from: an assessment of the global status of cause of death data. *Bulletin of the World Health Organization,* 2005, 83:171–177.
18. Shibuya K. Counting the dead is essential for health. *Bulletin of the World Health Organization,* 2006, 84:170–171.
19. *WHO mortality database: tables* [online database]. Geneva, World Health Organization, 2007 (http://www.who.int/healthinfo/morttables/en/index.html, accessed 4 April 2007).
20. *WHO survey data centre: World Health Survey.* Geneva, World Health Organization, 2007 (http://surveydata.who.int/, accessed 4 April 2007).
21. *Revised global burden of disease (GBD) 2002 estimates.* Geneva, World Health Organization, 2005 (http://www.who.int/healthinfo/bodgbd2002revised/en/index.html, accessed 4 April 2007).
22. Hosseinpoor AR et al. Decomposing socioeconomic inequality in infant mortality in Iran. *International Journal of Epidemiology,* 2006, 35:1211–1219.
23. *A WHO report on inequities in maternal and child health in Mozambique.* Geneva, World Health Organization, 2007.
24. *Global tuberculosis control: surveillance, planning, financing. WHO report 2007.* Geneva, World Health Organization, 2007 (WHO/HTM/TB/2007.376).
25. *The Global Plan to Stop TB 2006–2015.* Geneva, Stop TB Partnership, World Health Organization, 2006 (WHO/HTM/STB/2006.35).
26. *National health accounts.* Geneva, World Health Organization, 2007 (http://www.who.int/nha, accessed 4 April 2007).

Part 2
World health statistics

Health status: mortality

Figures have been computed by WHO to ensure comparability; thus they are not necessarily the official statistics of Member States, which may use alternative rigorous methods.

	Member State	WHO region	Life expectancy at birth[a] (years)		Healthy life expectancy (HALE) at birth[b] (years)		Probability of dying aged 15–60 years[a] per 1 000 population (adult mortality rate)		Probability of dying aged < 5 years per 1 000 live births[a] (under-5 mortality rate)	Infant mortality rate[a] (per 1 000 live births)	Neonatal mortality rate[c] (per 1 000 live births)	Maternal mortality ratio[d] (per 100 000 live births)
			Male	Female	Male	Female	Male	Female	Both sexes	Both sexes	Both sexes	Female
			2005	2005	2002	2002	2005	2005	2005	2005	2004	2000
1	Afghanistan	EMR	42	42	35	36	504	448	257	165	60	1 900
2	Albania	EUR	69	73	59	63	167	98	18	16	9	55
3	Algeria	AFR	70	72	60	62	151	123	39	34	22	140
4	Andorra	EUR	77	84	70	75	107	45	6	6	2	...
5	Angola	AFR	39	41	32	35	583	512	260	154	54	1 700
6	Antigua and Barbuda	AMR	70	75	60	64	189	117	12	11	8	...
7	Argentina	AMR	72	78	62	68	162	86	16	14	10	70
8	Armenia	EUR	65	72	59	63	249	109	29	26	18	55
9	Australia	WPR	79	84	71	74	84	47	6	5	3	6
10	Austria	EUR	77	82	69	74	111	55	5	4	3	5
11	Azerbaijan	EUR	64	67	56	59	187	121	89	74	35	94
12	Bahamas	AMR	70	76	61	66	254	142	15	13	5	60
13	Bahrain	EMR	73	76	64	64	111	75	11	9	4	33
14	Bangladesh	SEAR	62	63	55	53	251	258	73	54	36	380
15	Barbados	AMR	71	78	63	68	192	104	12	11	8	95
16	Belarus	EUR	63	75	57	65	366	133	9	7	3	36
17	Belgium	EUR	76	82	69	73	120	64	5	4	2	10
18	Belize	AMR	67	74	58	62	244	135	17	15	17	140
19	Benin	AFR	52	53	43	45	394	358	150	89	36	850
20	Bhutan	SEAR	62	65	53	53	250	190	75	65	30	420
21	Bolivia	AMR	63	67	54	55	245	180	65	52	24	420
22	Bosnia and Herzegovina	EUR	70	77	62	66	186	88	15	13	10	31
23	Botswana	AFR	42	41	36	35	758	750	120	86	46	100
24	Brazil	AMR	68	75	57	62	225	118	33	28	13	260
25	Brunei Darussalam	WPR	76	79	65	66	103	77	9	8	4	37
26	Bulgaria	EUR	69	76	63	67	213	92	15	12	7	32
27	Burkina Faso	AFR	48	49	35	36	428	388	191	96	32	1 000
28	Burundi	AFR	46	48	33	37	481	419	190	114	41	1 000
29	Cambodia	WPR	51	57	46	49	429	297	143	98	48	450
30	Cameroon	AFR	50	51	41	42	444	434	149	87	30	730
31	Canada	AMR	78	83	70	74	90	56	6	5	3	5
32	Cape Verde	AFR	67	72	59	63	288	132	35	26	9	150
33	Central African Republic	AFR	42	42	37	38	613	605	193	115	52	1 100
34	Chad	AFR	46	48	40	42	466	407	208	124	42	1 100
35	Chile	AMR	74	81	65	70	128	64	10	8	5	30
36	China	WPR	71	74	63	65	155	98	27	23	18	56
37	Colombia	AMR	71	78	58	66	179	87	21	17	13	130
38	Comoros	AFR	62	67	54	55	252	180	71	53	25	480
39	Congo	AFR	54	55	45	47	430	398	108	79	30	510
40	Cook Islands	WPR	70	75	61	63	153	102	20	17	10	...
41	Costa Rica	AMR	75	80	65	69	125	73	12	11	8	25
42	Côte d'Ivoire	AFR	42	47	38	41	573	497	196	118	64	690
43	Croatia	EUR	72	79	64	69	166	65	7	6	5	10
44	Cuba	AMR	75	79	67	70	128	83	7	5	4	33
45	Cyprus	EUR	77	82	67	68	94	45	5	4	2	47

Cause-specific mortality rate (per 100 000 population)			Age-standardized mortality rate by cause[h,i] (per 100 000 population)				Distribution of YLL by broader causes[h,j,k] (%)			Distribution of causes of death among children aged < 5 years[k,m] (%)							
HIV/AIDS[a]	TB among HIV-negative people[l]	TB among HIV-positive people[l]	Non-communicable diseases	Cardio-vascular diseases	Cancer	Injuries	Communicable diseases[l]	Non-communicable diseases	Injuries	Neonatal diseases	HIV/AIDS	Diarrhoeal diseases	Measles	Malaria	Pneumonia	Injuries	Other
Both sexes			Both sexes				Both sexes			Both sexes							
2005	2005	2005	2002	2002	2002	2002	2002	2002	2002	2000	2000	2000	2000	2000	2000	2000	2000
<10	35	<1	1 269	706	153	134	76	18	6	26.0	0.3	18.9	5.9	1.0	24.8	1.1	22.1
...	3	...	814	537	154	64	17	63	20	52.8	0.0	10.5	0.1	0.4	10.6	4.4	21.2
<10	2	<1	598	314	103	85	50	30	20	48.0	0.0	11.9	0.9	0.5	13.7	5.0	20.0
...	2	...	369	125	126	31	6	80	14	...	...	...	...	...	...	...	...
188	27	9	982	486	179	231	84	8	8	22.2	2.2	19.1	4.8	8.3	24.8	1.4	17.2
...	<1	...	717	343	144	35	21	69	10	25.3	1.0	2.4	0.0	0.0	1.5	2.4	67.4
11	5	<1	521	212	142	52	18	66	17	56.5	0.2	1.3	0.0	0.0	3.4	7.7	30.8
<50	10	<1	800	498	146	39	13	78	9	48.4	0.2	10.5	0.1	0.5	11.8	5.8	22.7
<10	<1	<1	362	140	127	35	5	77	17	55.6	0.0	0.1	0.0	0.0	1.2	10.6	32.5
<10	1	<1	406	204	127	38	3	83	14	56.0	0.0	0.0	0.0	0.0	0.7	8.4	34.9
<10	10	<1	892	613	113	29	36	58	6	44.1	0.0	15.3	0.1	1.0	18.4	1.3	19.7
<200	5	1	490	222	112	73	35	45	20	43.5	5.3	0.8	0.0	0.0	5.3	13.0	32.1
...	4	<1	746	312	127	37	10	68	22	46.0	0.2	0.7	0.0	0.0	1.4	10.2	41.5
<10	47	<1	762	428	111	101	60	28	12	45.4	0.0	20.0	2.0	0.7	17.6	2.7	11.4
<200	1	<1	535	245	135	30	26	65	10	63.8	1.7	0.0	0.0	0.0	0.0	1.7	32.8
...	8	<1	839	592	143	154	7	68	25	37.5	3.2	1.5	0.0	0.0	9.0	18.1	30.8
<10	1	<1	427	162	148	45	5	80	15	50.1	0.5	0.3	0.0	0.0	0.8	9.7	38.7
<200	4	<1	651	317	147	79	40	41	19	49.0	1.0	3.5	0.0	0.0	6.9	9.8	29.9
114	14	2	852	432	154	116	82	10	8	25.0	2.2	17.1	5.3	27.2	21.1	2.1	0.0
<10	19	<1	771	441	112	112	65	25	10	38.9	0.7	20.9	1.2	0.8	18.8	2.4	16.3
<10	31	<1	824	260	256	80	55	34	11	37.9	0.1	14.3	0.1	0.7	17.1	5.1	24.7
...	8	...	699	492	121	43	7	81	13	52.7	0.0	0.6	0.0	0.0	2.5	3.7	40.5
1 020	39	48	653	338	124	72	93	4	3	40.3	53.8	1.1	0.1	0.0	1.4	3.3	0.0
8	7	1	712	341	142	81	30	50	20	38.0	0.3	12.0	0.0	0.5	13.2	3.2	32.8
<50	5	<1	517	210	114	33	16	63	21	63.7	0.0	1.1	0.0	0.0	0.7	9.2	25.4
...	5	...	756	554	125	42	5	87	9	47.3	0.0	2.3	0.0	0.0	16.1	5.2	29.1
91	50	9	901	459	162	149	87	7	7	18.3	4.0	18.8	3.4	20.3	23.3	1.5	10.4
172	65	18	843	439	146	301	81	7	12	23.3	8.0	18.2	3.0	8.4	22.8	1.8	14.6
114	81	6	853	392	148	72	72	22	6	29.8	2.0	16.6	2.3	0.9	20.6	1.7	26.1
282	15	8	848	436	150	118	81	11	8	24.8	7.2	17.3	4.1	22.8	21.5	2.2	0.0
<10	<1	<1	388	141	138	34	6	80	15	58.5	0.0	0.2	0.0	0.0	1.1	7.2	32.9
...	37	...	692	356	127	39	51	37	12	25.9	3.7	12.2	4.4	4.3	13.3	3.5	32.6
594	48	43	863	445	154	146	84	9	7	27.2	12.4	14.7	6.5	18.5	18.7	2.0	0.0
113	54	16	869	443	156	131	85	8	7	24.0	4.1	18.1	7.0	22.3	22.8	1.8	0.1
<10	1	<1	453	165	137	50	17	64	19	52.8	0.1	0.5	0.0	0.0	6.2	9.1	31.2
2	15	<1	665	291	148	79	23	56	21	49.2	0.1	11.8	0.4	0.4	13.4	8.4	16.3
18	7	<1	511	240	117	141	25	35	40	62.1	1.4	10.3	0.0	0.2	10.4	4.6	11.0
<50	7	<1	736	381	128	83	70	18	12	37.3	3.7	13.6	5.9	19.4	16.3	3.4	0.5
275	51	18	762	393	134	147	79	11	11	30.9	9.3	11.2	6.6	25.7	13.6	2.6	0.0
...	3	...	616	326	69	38	29	57	13	96.1	0.0	0.7	0.5	0.0	1.1	0.2	1.4
<10	1	<1	457	185	125	55	22	57	21	58.7	0.2	3.0	0.0	0.0	4.0	3.9	30.1
358	69	30	873	436	160	179	78	11	10	34.9	5.6	14.8	2.5	20.5	19.6	2.2	0.0
...	6	...	613	356	167	48	5	84	11	65.3	0.0	0.3	0.0	0.0	1.3	8.5	24.6
<10	<1	<1	435	215	129	54	10	73	17	49.9	0.0	1.3	0.0	0.0	4.1	7.9	36.9
...	<1	...	530	354	94	33	12	74	14	61.5	0.1	3.2	0.0	0.0	1.7	5.4	28.2

Health status: mortality

Figures have been computed by WHO to ensure comparability; thus they are not necessarily the official statistics of Member States, which may use alternative rigorous methods.

	Member State	WHO region	Life expectancy at birth[a] (years)		Healthy life expectancy (HALE) at birth[b] (years)		Probability of dying aged 15–60 years[a] per 1 000 population (adult mortality rate)		Probability of dying aged < 5 years per 1 000 live births[a] (under-5 mortality rate)	Infant mortality rate[a] (per 1 000 live births)	Neonatal mortality rate[c] (per 1 000 live births)	Maternal mortality ratio[d] (per 100 000 live births)
			Male	Female	Male	Female	Male	Female	Both sexes	Both sexes	Both sexes	Female
			2005	2005	2002	2002	2005	2005	2005	2005	2004	2000
46	Czech Republic	EUR	73	79	66	71	156	70	4	3	2	9
47	Democratic People's Republic of Korea	SEAR	65	68	58	60	231	168	55	42	22	67
48	Democratic Republic of the Congo	AFR	44	48	35	39	501	425	205	129	47	990
49	Denmark	EUR	76	80	69	71	116	70	5	4	3	7
50	Djibouti	EMR	53	56	43	43	384	336	133	88	45	730
51	Dominica	AMR	72	76	62	66	192	111	15	13	10	...
52	Dominican Republic	AMR	65	72	57	62	254	138	31	26	18	150
53	Ecuador	AMR	70	75	60	64	205	124	25	22	13	130
54	Egypt	EMR	66	70	58	60	237	155	33	28	17	84
55	El Salvador	AMR	69	74	57	62	229	123	27	23	12	150
56	Equatorial Guinea	AFR	45	47	45	46	484	438	205	123	47	880
57	Eritrea	AFR	59	63	49	51	337	271	78	50	21	630
58	Estonia	EUR	67	78	59	69	281	100	7	6	4	38
59	Ethiopia	AFR	50	53	41	42	413	348	164	109	41	850
60	Fiji	WPR	66	72	57	61	265	166	18	16	10	75
61	Finland	EUR	76	82	69	74	136	62	4	3	2	5
62	France	EUR	77	84	69	75	128	58	5	4	2	17
63	Gabon	AFR	54	57	50	53	440	406	91	59	31	420
64	Gambia	AFR	53	57	48	51	367	301	137	97	44	540
65	Georgia	EUR	68	75	62	67	180	69	45	41	25	32
66	Germany	EUR	76	82	70	74	110	57	5	4	3	9
67	Ghana	AFR	56	58	49	50	355	322	112	68	43	540
68	Greece	EUR	77	82	69	73	110	47	5	4	3	10
69	Grenada	AMR	66	70	58	60	253	216	21	17	11	...
70	Guatemala	AMR	65	71	55	60	295	166	43	32	19	240
71	Guinea	AFR	53	55	44	46	367	334	150	98	39	740
72	Guinea-Bissau	AFR	46	48	40	41	483	423	200	124	47	1 100
73	Guyana	AMR	63	64	53	57	265	249	63	47	22	170
74	Haiti	AMR	53	56	43	44	415	335	120	83	32	680
75	Honduras	AMR	65	70	56	61	266	161	40	31	17	110
76	Hungary	EUR	69	77	62	68	256	107	8	6	5	11
77	Iceland	EUR	79	83	72	74	73	50	3	2	1	...
78	India	SEAR	62	64	53	54	280	207	74	56	39	540
79	Indonesia	SEAR	66	69	57	59	234	196	36	28	17	230
80	Iran (Islamic Republic of)	EMR	68	73	56	59	180	112	36	31	19	76
81	Iraq	EMR	...	...[n]	49	51	...	...[n]	...[n]	...[n]	63	250
82	Ireland	EUR	77	81	68	72	91	57	5	4	4	4
83	Israel	EUR	78	82	70	72	91	50	5	4	3	13
84	Italy	EUR	78	84	71	75	89	46	4	4	3	5
85	Jamaica	AMR	70	74	64	66	182	117	20	17	10	87
86	Japan	WPR	79	86	72	78	92	45	4	3	1	10
87	Jordan	EMR	69	73	60	62	186	119	26	22	16	41
88	Kazakhstan	EUR	58	69	53	59	437	194	31	27	32	210
89	Kenya	AFR	51	51	44	45	464	483	120	78	34	1 000
90	Kiribati	WPR	62	68	52	56	296	173	65	48	25	...

World Health Statistics 2007

Cause-specific mortality rate (per 100 000 population)			Age-standardized mortality rate by cause[h,i] (per 100 000 population)				Distribution of YLL by broader causes[h,i,k] (%)			Distribution of causes of death among children aged < 5 years[k,m] (%)							
HIV/AIDS[a]	TB among HIV-negative people[i]	TB among HIV-positive people[n]	Non-communicable diseases	Cardio-vascular diseases	Cancer	Injuries	Communicable diseases[i]	Non-communicable diseases	Injuries	Neonatal diseases	HIV/AIDS	Diarrhoeal diseases	Measles	Malaria	Pneumonia	Injuries	Other
Both sexes			Both sexes				Both sexes			Both sexes							
2005	2005	2005	2002	2002	2002	2002	2002	2002	2002	2000	2000	2000	2000	2000	2000	2000	2000
<10	1	<1	568	315	177	50	3	83	13	48.9	0.0	0.2	0.0	0.0	3.6	12.5	34.7
...	13	...	691	371	102	65	44	46	11	41.8	0.7	18.9	0.8	0.7	15.2	3.0	18.9
156	57	17	909	465	161	273	82	7	11	25.7	3.7	18.1	4.7	16.9	23.1	1.6	6.3
<10	<1	<1	503	182	167	40	4	86	10	73.8	0.0	0.3	0.0	0.0	0.9	5.5	19.4
151	106	22	926	533	116	92	76	17	8	27.0	2.7	16.6	4.4	0.8	20.4	1.8	26.2
...	3	...	590	257	144	45	19	68	13	99.9	0.0	0.0	0.0	0.0	0.0	0.0	0.1
75	13	1	687	381	131	59	56	33	12	47.2	3.9	11.7	0.1	0.6	13.0	2.9	20.6
12	26	<1	576	244	129	89	37	42	21	47.2	1.1	11.0	0.1	0.5	12.0	4.6	20.9
<10	3	<1	959	560	84	35	32	61	8	44.3	0.0	12.8	0.1	0.4	14.6	2.1	25.7
36	8	<1	557	223	102	101	41	38	21	39.9	1.7	12.4	0.0	0.5	13.4	3.7	28.4
<200	36	11	864	438	155	144	79	12	9	27.5	7.4	13.6	7.4	24.0	17.3	2.5	0.3
127	59	10	762	398	133	92	81	11	8	27.4	6.2	15.6	2.5	13.6	18.6	3.0	13.0
...	6	<1	674	435	150	144	6	67	27	54.3	0.0	1.4	0.0	0.0	2.1	17.9	24.3
...	64	9	859	435	147	104	82	12	6	30.2	3.8	17.3	4.2	6.1	22.3	1.7	14.3
<50	4	<1	825	470	86	40	27	63	10	41.2	0.2	10.6	0.0	0.0	9.2	2.9	36.0
<10	<1	<1	422	201	115	60	5	76	20	55.1	0.0	0.8	0.0	0.0	1.2	6.9	36.0
2	1	<1	368	118	142	48	6	78	16	52.6	0.0	0.9	0.0	0.0	0.6	8.3	37.5
340	41	24	813	410	158	103	72	18	9	35.1	10.1	8.8	4.4	28.3	10.7	2.5	0.0
86	39	7	805	413	144	109	75	15	10	36.6	1.3	12.2	2.5	29.4	15.5	2.6	0.0
<50	11	<1	745	584	91	25	13	81	6	52.1	0.0	11.5	0.1	0.3	12.5	1.2	22.3
<10	<1	<1	444	211	141	29	5	86	10	50.7	0.1	0.2	0.0	0.0	0.7	6.6	41.8
131	41	7	786	404	138	97	74	16	10	28.5	5.7	12.2	2.9	33.0	14.6	3.0	0.0
<10	2	<1	457	258	132	35	4	83	13	63.0	0.0	0.0	0.0	0.0	2.6	5.8	28.6
...	<1	...	870	448	199	51	23	66	10	43.8	2.6	1.6	0.0	0.0	9.5	5.2	37.3
21	12	<1	562	188	93	98	60	27	13	37.3	2.7	13.1	0.1	0.4	15.0	1.5	29.8
76	46	6	853	432	156	147	80	11	9	28.8	2.3	16.5	5.5	24.5	20.9	1.4	0.0
170	31	9	883	449	159	138	86	8	6	24.1	2.6	18.6	3.4	21.0	23.4	1.4	5.5
160	22	4	822	526	86	97	56	30	14	33.7	7.7	21.4	0.0	0.7	5.2	6.2	25.2
188	51	7	786	402	112	38	84	15	2	26.4	8.3	16.5	0.5	0.7	20.2	0.4	27.0
51	11	1	758	348	139	66	52	35	13	43.1	6.3	12.2	0.0	0.4	13.8	4.2	20.1
...	3	<1	695	364	201	67	3	85	12	56.9	0.0	0.1	0.0	0.0	3.9	5.6	33.6
<50	<1	<1	385	164	136	34	5	77	17	61.0	0.0	0.0	0.0	0.0	0.0	4.9	34.1
...	27	2	750	428	109	117	58	29	13	45.2	0.7	20.3	3.7	0.9	18.5	2.2	8.5
2	41	<1	727	361	132	87	41	44	15	37.6	0.0	18.3	4.7	0.5	14.4	2.8	21.8
2	3	<1	742	466	113	133	22	49	28	62.9	0.1	5.5	0.0	0.2	6.4	12.8	12.1
...	11	<1	855	508	112	141	57	28	15	50.8	0.3	13.2	0.5	0.7	17.6	5.7	11.2
<10	1	<1	484	214	151	35	8	78	14	61.1	0.0	0.0	0.5	0.0	1.3	2.9	34.2
...	<1	...	399	136	133	30	9	76	14	52.8	0.0	0.6	0.0	0.0	0.4	5.9	40.3
5	<1	<1	403	174	134	29	5	86	10	62.0	0.2	0.0	0.0	0.0	1.0	4.0	32.8
49	<1	<1	672	326	151	12	30	66	4	52.1	6.1	9.6	0.0	0.0	9.3	2.4	20.6
1	3	<1	287	106	119	39	8	76	16	40.0	0.0	0.4	0.2	0.0	3.9	11.6	43.9
...	<1	<1	703	384	144	102	31	45	23	55.4	0.1	10.7	0.0	0.3	11.7	2.3	19.5
<10	19	<1	1 052	713	167	160	16	60	24	43.1	0.0	14.5	0.1	0.8	16.9	6.8	17.9
409	95	44	782	401	139	95	81	11	8	24.2	14.6	16.5	3.2	13.6	19.9	2.7	5.3
...	49	...	773	273	52	22	45	52	3	22.1	0.0	21.9	2.6	0.7	11.5	1.3	39.9

Health status: mortality

Figures have been computed by WHO to ensure comparability; thus they are not necessarily the official statistics of Member States, which may use alternative rigorous methods.

	Member State	WHO region	Life expectancy at birth[a] (years)		Healthy life expectancy (HALE) at birth[b] (years)		Probability of dying aged 15–60 years[a] per 1 000 population (adult mortality rate)		Probability of dying aged < 5 years per 1 000 live births[a] (under-5 mortality rate)	Infant mortality rate[a] (per 1 000 live births)	Neonatal mortality rate[c] (per 1 000 live births)	Maternal mortality ratio[d] (per 100 000 live births)
			Male	Female	Male	Female	Male	Female	Both sexes	Both sexes	Both sexes	Female
			2005	2005	2002	2002	2005	2005	2005	2005	2004	2000
91	Kuwait	EMR	77	79	67	67	71	54	12	10	7	12
92	Kyrgyzstan	EUR	61	68	52	58	311	165	67	58	30	110
93	Lao People's Democratic Republic	WPR	59	61	47	47	327	297	79	62	30	650
94	Latvia	EUR	65	76	58	68	314	114	10	8	6	61
95	Lebanon	EMR	68	73	59	62	195	135	30	27	19	150
96	Lesotho	AFR	42	41	30	33	721	732	132	102	52	550
97	Liberia	AFR	41	44	34	37	536	470	235	157	66	760
98	Libyan Arab Jamahiriya	EMR	70	75	62	65	185	108	19	18	11	97
99	Lithuania	EUR	65	77	59	68	326	109	9	7	5	19
100	Luxembourg	EUR	76	82	69	74	119	53	5	4	3	28
101	Madagascar	AFR	56	60	47	50	318	240	119	74	41	550
102	Malawi	AFR	47	46	35	35	599	602	125	78	26	1 800
103	Malaysia	WPR	69	74	62	65	199	107	12	10	5	41
104	Maldives	SEAR	67	69	59	57	179	132	42	33	24	110
105	Mali	AFR	45	47	37	38	475	409	218	120	54	1 200
106	Malta	EUR	77	81	70	73	77	48	6	5	3	...
107	Marshall Islands	WPR	60	64	54	56	320	269	58	51	24	...
108	Mauritania	AFR	55	60	43	46	329	255	125	78	40	1 000
109	Mauritius	AFR	69	76	60	65	213	110	15	13	9	24
110	Mexico	AMR	72	77	63	68	162	94	27	22	11	83
111	Micronesia (Federated States of)	WPR	67	70	57	58	198	166	42	34	11	...
112	Monaco	EUR	78	85	71	75	104	45	4	3	2	...
113	Mongolia	WPR	62	69	53	58	304	183	49	39	18	110
114	Montenegro	EUR	71	77	...	...	176	85	10	9	...	...
115	Morocco	EMR	69	73	59	61	156	101	40	36	24	220
116	Mozambique	AFR	46	45	36	38	597	595	145	100	35	1 000
117	Myanmar	SEAR	56	62	50	53	350	237	104	74	49	360
118	Namibia	AFR	52	52	43	44	579	589	62	46	20	300
119	Nauru	WPR	58	65	53	57	448	303	30	25	14	...
120	Nepal	SEAR	61	61	52	51	295	283	74	56	32	740
121	Netherlands	EUR	77	81	70	73	89	65	5	4	3	16
122	New Zealand	WPR	77	82	69	72	92	61	6	5	3	7
123	Nicaragua	AMR	68	73	60	63	213	133	37	30	16	230
124	Niger	AFR	42	41	36	35	502	478	256	150	41	1 600
125	Nigeria	AFR	47	48	41	42	461	421	194	101	47	800
126	Niue	WPR	68	74	59	62	174	138	38	30	16	...
127	Norway	EUR	77	82	70	74	91	56	4	3	2	10
128	Oman	EMR	71	77	63	65	163	91	12	10	5	87
129	Pakistan	EMR	61	62	54	52	232	212	100	80	53	500
130	Palau	WPR	68	72	59	60	231	226	11	10	13	...
131	Panama	AMR	74	78	64	68	136	81	24	19	11	160
132	Papua New Guinea	WPR	59	63	51	52	325	270	74	54	32	300
133	Paraguay	AMR	70	76	60	64	169	105	23	20	12	170
134	Peru	AMR	70	74	60	62	178	129	27	23	11	410
135	Philippines	WPR	64	71	57	62	284	164	33	25	15	200

Cause-specific mortality rate (per 100 000 population)			Age-standardized mortality rate by cause[h,i] (per 100 000 population)				Distribution of YLL by broader causes[h,i,k] (%)			Distribution of causes of death among children aged < 5 years[k,m] (%)							
HIV/AIDS[s]	TB among HIV-negative people[f]	TB among HIV-positive people[g]	Non-communicable diseases	Cardio-vascular diseases	Cancer	Injuries	Communicable diseases	Non-communicable diseases	Injuries	Neonatal diseases	HIV/AIDS	Diarrhoeal diseases	Measles	Malaria	Pneumonia	Injuries	Other
Both sexes			Both sexes				Both sexes			Both sexes							
2005	2005	2005	2002	2002	2002	2002	2002	2002	2002	2000	2000	2000	2000	2000	2000	2000	2000
...	2	...	512	309	78	34	18	60	22	35.5	0.0	0.7	0.0	0.0	4.4	7.9	51.5
<10	17	<1	924	602	106	90	35	51	14	43.8	0.0	14.1	0.1	0.9	16.7	6.6	17.9
<10	24	<1	904	476	150	142	71	19	10	34.5	0.0	15.6	5.9	0.7	19.1	2.3	21.9
<50	9	<1	733	482	156	132	7	70	23	53.2	0.0	0.0	0.0	0.0	1.2	11.3	34.3
<10	1	<1	742	453	90	98	18	60	22	64.9	0.0	1.0	0.0	0.0	1.1	11.0	22.0
1 282	47	61	785	404	139	88	90	7	3	32.8	56.2	3.9	0.1	0.0	4.7	2.2	0.0
...	54	16	955	485	169	270	83	7	10	29.1	3.6	17.3	6.0	18.9	23.0	1.7	0.3
...	1	<1	650	411	79	55	31	53	16	55.6	0.1	8.4	0.1	0.0	8.5	2.6	24.8
<10	7	<1	640	391	161	136	4	68	28	41.4	0.0	0.3	0.0	0.0	5.3	17.4	35.6
<50	1	<1	406	177	134	51	5	76	19	54.0	0.0	0.0	0.0	0.0	1.1	14.9	29.9
16	43	2	837	430	147	112	79	12	9	25.6	1.3	16.9	5.0	20.1	20.7	2.4	8.0
605	49	49	835	430	150	105	89	6	5	21.7	14.0	18.1	0.3	14.1	22.6	1.7	7.6
16	15	<1	625	274	139	50	26	58	16	61.8	1.4	5.4	0.9	0.1	4.0	7.7	18.7
...	3	...	864	484	123	70	55	36	9	45.1	0.7	20.3	0.1	0.6	17.5	2.5	13.1
81	62	9	909	456	166	145	86	8	6	25.9	1.6	18.3	6.1	16.9	23.9	1.4	5.9
<50	<1	<1	429	214	124	24	8	83	9	66.7	0.0	0.0	0.0	0.0	0.0	6.0	27.4
...	32	...	997	526	125	62	31	59	10	37.1	0.3	14.1	0.5	0.0	13.5	3.1	31.4
<50	65	3	884	451	158	138	79	12	9	39.4	0.3	16.2	1.7	12.2	22.3	1.9	5.9
<10	11	<1	701	434	79	42	11	75	13	66.0	0.0	1.2	0.0	0.0	3.9	5.2	23.6
6	2	<1	503	163	88	58	27	54	19	52.5	0.1	5.1	0.0	0.0	8.5	7.0	26.8
...	14	...	782	410	93	39	40	51	9	49.2	0.3	8.0	1.5	0.0	11.3	2.7	26.9
...	<1	...	325	115	120	41	7	77	16	...	...	...	...	...	...	...	...
<10	23	<1	968	488	306	96	37	47	16	34.1	0.3	14.5	0.3	1.0	17.1	4.4	28.3
...	5	<1	...	...	...	...	...	...	...	...	...	...	...	...	...	...	...
4	7	<1	675	411	67	48	44	44	12	44.7	0.3	12.2	0.2	0.4	14.0	4.0	24.1
707	58	66	720	371	124	66	91	7	2	29.0	12.9	16.5	0.3	18.9	21.2	1.0	0.1
73	14	<1	796	432	115	105	60	29	11	39.1	0.9	21.1	2.4	9.0	19.3	2.0	6.2
837	42	35	754	385	146	93	83	10	6	38.5	53.0	2.5	0.1	0.0	3.0	3.0	0.0
...	18	...	1 137	666	138	132	19	68	13	7.0	0.0	37.8	5.5	0.0	30.3	19.4	0.1
19	22	<1	796	436	118	108	64	25	11	43.5	0.2	20.5	2.7	0.8	18.5	2.3	11.5
<10	<1	<1	443	171	155	23	7	85	8	63.1	0.0	0.0	0.0	0.0	1.1	5.2	30.6
...	<1	...	423	175	139	37	5	79	17	48.3	0.0	0.2	0.0	0.0	2.7	11.4	37.4
<10	7	<1	655	305	120	73	46	36	17	42.4	0.5	12.2	0.0	0.4	13.7	3.0	27.7
54	32	3	916	456	169	163	87	7	6	16.7	0.6	19.8	7.3	14.3	25.1	1.4	14.8
167	57	19	889	452	157	132	83	10	7	26.1	5.0	15.7	6.3	24.1	20.1	1.9	0.8
...	9	...	637	339	74	39	33	55	12	...	...	...	...	...	...	...	...
<10	<1	<1	416	181	137	35	5	83	12	54.0	0.0	0.3	0.0	0.0	1.4	6.2	38.1
...	<1	<1	688	409	105	41	24	57	19	42.3	0.3	8.1	0.0	0.1	7.2	4.1	37.9
2	37	<1	743	425	107	99	70	21	8	55.7	0.0	14.0	2.4	0.7	19.3	2.1	5.7
...	7	...	744	396	92	39	28	63	10	47.0	0.3	9.7	0.7	0.0	12.4	2.5	27.4
<50	3	<1	430	182	108	49	38	44	18	42.4	2.4	10.7	0.0	0.2	10.8	3.8	29.6
56	43	3	815	442	118	104	64	25	11	35.4	0.3	15.3	2.1	0.8	18.5	2.3	25.4
<10	12	<1	598	291	141	57	45	39	16	53.5	0.2	10.7	0.1	0.3	11.9	3.8	19.6
20	20	<1	584	190	175	69	43	42	15	38.5	0.9	12.2	0.0	0.4	13.6	9.5	24.9
<10	47	<1	642	336	91	58	45	42	13	36.9	0.0	12.0	1.2	0.4	13.4	2.7	33.5

Health status: mortality

Figures have been computed by WHO to ensure comparability; thus they are not necessarily the official statistics of Member States, which may use alternative rigorous methods.

	Member State	WHO region	Life expectancy at birth[a] (years)		Healthy life expectancy (HALE) at birth[b] (years)		Probability of dying aged 15–60 years[a] per 1 000 population (adult mortality rate)		Probability of dying aged < 5 years per 1 000 live births[a] (under-5 mortality rate)	Infant mortality rate[a] (per 1 000 live births)	Neonatal mortality rate[c] (per 1 000 live births)	Maternal mortality ratio[d] (per 100 000 live births)
			Male	Female	Male	Female	Male	Female	Both sexes	Both sexes	Both sexes	Female
			2005	2005	2002	2002	2005	2005	2005	2005	2004	2000
136	Poland	EUR	71	79	63	68	208	79	8	6	5	10
137	Portugal	EUR	75	81	67	72	139	59	5	4	3	8
138	Qatar	EMR	77	78	67	64	70	66	12	10	4	7
139	Republic of Korea	WPR	75	82	65	71	123	50	6	6	4	20
140	Republic of Moldova	EUR	65	72	57	62	301	141	16	14	12	36
141	Romania	EUR	68	76	61	65	230	102	19	16	10	58
142	Russian Federation	EUR	59	72	53	64	470	173	14	11	7	65
143	Rwanda	AFR	44	47	36	40	513	444	203	118	48	1 400
144	Saint Kitts and Nevis	AMR	69	72	60	63	197	145	20	18	11	...
145	Saint Lucia	AMR	72	78	61	64	204	106	14	13	11	...
146	Saint Vincent and the Grenadines	AMR	66	74	60	62	293	167	20	17	13	...
147	Samoa	WPR	66	70	59	60	235	203	29	24	14	...
148	San Marino	EUR	80	84	71	76	64	33	3	3	2	...
149	Sao Tome and Principe	AFR	57	60	54	55	301	236	118	75	38	...
150	Saudi Arabia	EMR	68	74	60	63	195	119	26	21	11	23
151	Senegal	AFR	54	57	47	49	345	285	136	77	35	690
152	Serbia	EUR	70	75	...	...	192	98	9	8	...	...
153	Seychelles	AFR	68	77	57	65	246	107	13	12	7	...
154	Sierra Leone	AFR	37	40	27	30	582	501	282	165	56	2 000
155	Singapore	WPR	78	82	69	71	83	48	3	2	1	15
156	Slovakia	EUR	70	78	63	69	201	77	9	7	4	10
157	Slovenia	EUR	74	81	67	72	152	67	4	3	2	17
158	Solomon Islands	WPR	68	72	55	57	190	141	29	24	23	130
159	Somalia	EMR	45	45	36	38	465	423	225	133	49	1 100
160	South Africa	AFR	50	52	43	45	598	532	68	51	17	230
161	Spain	EUR	77	84	70	75	111	46	5	4	2	5
162	Sri Lanka	SEAR	68	75	59	64	228	118	14	12	8	92
163	Sudan	EMR	57	62	47	50	357	268	90	62	27	590
164	Suriname	AMR	66	71	57	61	225	144	39	30	17	110
165	Swaziland	AFR	38	37	33	35	793	794	160	104	40	370
166	Sweden	EUR	79	83	72	75	78	50	4	3	2	8
167	Switzerland	EUR	79	84	71	75	84	46	5	4	3	7
168	Syrian Arab Republic	EMR	70	75	60	63	184	124	15	14	7	160
169	Tajikistan	EUR	64	66	53	56	192	167	71	59	38	100
170	Thailand	SEAR	67	73	58	62	265	155	21	18	9	44
171	The former Yugoslav Republic of Macedonia	EUR	71	76	62	65	164	77	17	15	9	13
172	Timor-Leste	SEAR	63	68	48	52	244	166	61	52	29	660
173	Togo	AFR	52	56	44	46	400	340	139	78	39	570
174	Tonga	WPR	72	70	62	62	126	201	24	20	12	...
175	Trinidad and Tobago	AMR	67	74	60	64	268	158	19	17	10	110
176	Tunisia	EMR	70	75	61	64	166	108	24	20	13	120
177	Turkey	EUR	69	74	61	63	181	112	29	26	16	70
178	Turkmenistan	EUR	57	65	52	57	321	164	104	81	37	31
179	Tuvalu	WPR	61	63	53	53	327	287	38	31	21	...
180	Uganda	AFR	48	51	42	44	506	457	136	79	30	880

WORLD HEALTH STATISTICS 2007

Cause-specific mortality rate (per 100 000 population)			Age-standardized mortality rate by cause[h,i] (per 100 000 population)				Distribution of YLL by broader causes[h,i,k] (%)			Distribution of causes of death among children aged < 5 years[k,m] (%)							
HIV/AIDS[a]	TB among HIV-negative people	TB among HIV-positive people[a]	Non-communicable diseases	Cardio-vascular diseases	Cancer	Injuries	Communicable diseases[l]	Non-communicable diseases	Injuries	Neonatal diseases	HIV/AIDS	Diarrhoeal diseases	Measles	Malaria	Pneumonia	Injuries	Other
Both sexes			Both sexes				Both sexes			Both sexes							
2005	2005	2005	2002	2002	2002	2002	2002	2002	2002	2000	2000	2000	2000	2000	2000	2000	2000
<10	4	<1	593	324	180	53	4	81	15	59.1	0.0	0.1	0.0	0.0	2.7	5.6	32.5
<10	3	<1	461	208	140	33	13	77	10	47.9	0.1	0.1	0.0	0.1	1.8	9.0	41.0
...	6	...	629	340	75	40	16	63	21	29.6	0.1	8.4	0.0	0.0	7.7	5.2	48.9
<10	11	<1	537	186	169	67	7	72	21	71.5	0.0	0.4	0.2	0.0	1.8	11.2	15.0
33	18	1	923	619	116	97	11	71	18	46.1	0.0	2.0	0.0	0.0	15.5	13.3	23.1
...	18	...	728	479	141	56	11	77	12	41.4	0.1	2.5	0.0	0.0	27.1	8.6	20.3
...	19	1	960	688	152	217	8	64	28	40.8	0.4	2.5	0.0	0.0	6.3	12.0	38.0
232	72	19	831	425	150	126	85	8	7	21.7	5.0	18.5	1.6	4.6	23.2	1.8	23.7
...	2	...	689	420	108	45	26	62	12	2.8	0.0	14.4	0.0	0.0	0.0	7.9	74.9
...	2	...	646	304	129	52	20	63	17	30.9	1.3	1.3	0.0	0.0	1.3	4.7	60.4
...	5	...	685	315	155	55	27	60	13	49.6	2.9	0.5	0.0	0.0	10.5	4.0	32.4
...	3	...	782	417	95	40	31	58	11	49.2	0.3	9.7	0.1	0.1	10.2	2.9	27.4
...	<1	...	380	223	140	22	5	85	10	...	...	...	...	...	...	...	...
...	27	...	764	396	133	87	67	21	12	32.1	3.7	16.0	4.8	0.6	21.2	3.5	18.1
...	5	...	701	405	109	72	22	53	25	40.2	0.1	6.2	0.0	0.2	6.6	14.5	32.2
45	51	4	832	426	146	125	76	13	11	22.8	1.0	17.1	8.1	27.6	20.7	2.6	0.2
...	5	<1	...	...	...	...	...	...	...	...	...	...	...	...	...	...	...
...	5	...	657	336	131	69	16	64	21	27.2	0.0	0.0	0.0	0.0	10.1	12.3	50.3
83	98	12	1 017	515	181	250	86	6	8	21.9	1.3	19.7	5.3	12.4	25.5	1.2	12.7
<10	2	<1	376	171	128	23	9	79	12	40.0	0.0	0.4	0.0	0.0	9.0	7.1	43.5
...	3	<1	636	371	170	50	4	81	14	52.7	0.0	1.4	0.0	0.0	9.4	6.0	30.5
<10	2	<1	503	228	160	59	4	80	17	64.4	0.0	0.0	0.0	0.0	0.0	5.9	29.7
...	23	...	786	409	90	37	49	44	7	49.5	0.3	8.8	0.5	0.1	9.5	2.5	28.7
50	38	2	1 086	580	143	235	76	14	11	23.3	0.8	18.7	6.8	4.5	23.9	2.6	19.5
675	30	41	808	410	154	120	77	15	8	35.1	57.1	0.8	0.0	0.0	0.9	5.0	1.1
5	3	<1	395	137	131	31	6	81	13	52.4	0.0	0.1	0.0	0.0	1.3	6.5	39.6
<10	8	<1	711	314	118	82	19	61	20	59.5	0.0	13.5	1.7	0.4	8.5	5.4	10.9
94	59	7	903	499	112	163	60	23	17	31.4	2.9	12.9	5.4	21.2	15.5	4.6	6.2
<200	12	2	781	421	133	86	37	45	18	40.5	2.5	13.1	0.3	2.4	11.5	5.8	23.9
1 550	107	197	732	364	162	72	91	5	4	26.8	47.0	9.6	0.2	0.2	11.8	3.8	0.5
<10	<1	<1	379	176	116	30	4	85	11	59.4	0.0	0.0	0.0	0.0	0.8	3.4	36.3
<10	<1	<1	358	142	116	32	5	82	13	62.1	0.0	0.2	0.0	0.0	0.7	7.5	29.5
...	4	...	728	410	60	49	30	56	15	42.7	0.0	9.6	0.0	0.2	9.9	3.4	34.1
<10	38	<1	1 036	753	90	64	49	41	10	29.7	0.0	16.4	0.2	0.8	19.9	2.6	30.4
33	17	2	559	199	129	74	43	40	17	44.9	6.2	16.2	0.1	0.3	11.5	4.8	16.0
<10	5	<1	745	504	145	74	8	72	20	63.1	0.0	5.0	0.0	0.0	4.3	2.5	25.1
...	88	...	814	441	118	112	63	26	11	32.3	0.7	21.9	3.5	0.4	19.6	1.9	19.7
148	81	20	831	427	147	117	79	12	9	29.0	5.8	13.8	6.6	25.3	17.1	2.5	0.0
...	3	...	684	363	85	29	29	62	9	57.2	0.0	10.0	1.8	1.3	7.3	2.0	20.4
146	1	<1	729	379	121	50	40	50	10	46.3	4.7	1.3	0.0	0.0	2.0	3.1	42.5
<10	3	...	685	417	78	72	18	63	19	52.7	0.0	7.0	0.0	0.2	7.6	9.7	22.8
...	5	...	757	542	95	42	31	56	13	49.1	0.0	12.2	0.3	0.5	14.0	4.0	19.8
...	10	<1	1 115	844	99	74	35	52	13	37.8	0.0	15.6	0.1	0.9	18.8	4.8	22.0
...	55	...	1 046	541	129	69	34	55	11	40.0	0.3	13.2	1.2	0.0	13.5	3.0	28.8
316	59	32	824	422	146	154	84	8	8	23.6	7.7	17.2	3.0	23.1	21.1	2.2	2.1

29

Health status: mortality

Figures have been computed by WHO to ensure comparability; thus they are not necessarily the official statistics of Member States, which may use alternative rigorous methods.

	Member State	WHO region	Life expectancy at birth[a] (years)		Healthy life expectancy (HALE) at birth[b] (years)		Probability of dying aged 15–60 years[a] per 1 000 population (adult mortality rate)		Probability of dying aged < 5 years per 1 000 live births[a] (under-5 mortality rate)	Infant mortality rate[a] (per 1 000 live births)	Neonatal mortality rate[c] (per 1 000 live births)	Maternal mortality ratio[d] (per 100 000 live births)
			Male	Female	Male	Female	Male	Female	Both sexes	Both sexes	Both sexes	Female
			2005	2005	2002	2002	2005	2005	2005	2005	2004	2000
181	Ukraine	EUR	61	73	55	64	403	150	17	13	7	38
182	United Arab Emirates	EMR	76	79	64	64	86	64	9	8	4	54
183	United Kingdom	EUR	77	81	69	72	101	62	6	5	3	11
184	United Republic of Tanzania	AFR	48	50	40	41	541	505	122	76	35	1 500
185	United States of America	AMR	75	80	67	71	137	81	8	7	4	14
186	Uruguay	AMR	71	79	63	69	166	88	15	13	7	20
187	Uzbekistan	EUR	63	69	58	61	236	143	68	57	26	24
188	Vanuatu	WPR	67	70	58	59	209	168	38	31	18	...
189	Venezuela (Bolivarian Republic of)	AMR	72	78	62	67	185	96	21	18	11	78
190	Viet Nam	WPR	69	74	60	63	195	119	19	16	12	130
191	Yemen	EMR	59	62	48	51	286	219	102	76	41	570
192	Zambia	AFR	40	40	35	35	702	666	182	104	40	750
193	Zimbabwe	AFR	43	42	34	33	771	789	86	60	36	1 100
194	The former state union of Serbia and Montenegro[e]	EUR	...	...	63	65	...	...	...	...	9	9

Region											
African Region	AFR	48	50	40	42	480	438	165	99	40	910
Region of the Americas	AMR	72	77	63	67	171	97	24	20	11	140
South-East Asia Region	SEAR	62	65	54	55	272	207	68	51	35	460
European Region	EUR	69	77	62	68	231	99	19	16	10	39
Eastern Mediterranean Region	EMR	62	64	53	54	242	189	90	66	38	460
Western Pacific Region	WPR	71	75	63	66	157	96	28	23	17	80
Global		64	68	56	59	233	164	74	51	28	400

... Data not available or not applicable; AFR, African Region; AMR, Region of the Americas; SEAR, South-East Asia Region; EUR, European Region; EMR, Eastern Mediterranean Region; WPR, Western Pacific Region.

The global values for rates and ratios are weighted averages; for absolute numbers they are the sums of all WHO regions.

[a] *Life tables for WHO Member States*. Geneva, World Health Organization, 2006 (http://www.who.int/whosis/database/life_tables/life_tables.cfm).

[b] *The World Health Report 2004: changing history*. Geneva, World Health Organization, 2004 (http://www.who.int/whr/2004/en/index.html.)

[c] *Updated estimates based on Neonatal and perinatal mortality: country, regional and global estimates*. Geneva, World Health Organization, 2006 (http://www.who.int/reproductive-health/docs/neonatal_perinatal_mortality/text.pdf).

[d] *Maternal mortality in 2000: estimates developed by WHO, UNICEF and UNFPA*. Geneva, World Health Organization, 2004 (http://www.who.int/reproductive-health/publications/maternal_mortality_2000/mme.pdf).

[e] *Based on 2006 report on the global AIDS epidemic*. Geneva, Joint United Nations Programme on HIV/AIDS, World Health Organization, 2006. See Annex 2: HIV and AIDS estimates and data, 2005 and 2003. Ranges of estimates are available from this document.

[f] These are classified as deaths from tuberculosis according to the *International Classification of Diseases, tenth revision* (A15–A19, B90). Geneva, World Health Organization, 1992. Source: *Global tuberculosis control: surveillance, planning, financing. WHO report 2007*. Geneva, World Health Organization, 2007 (WHO/HTM/TB/2007.376) (http://www.who.int/tb/publications/global_report).

[g] These deaths are classified as HIV disease resulting in tuberculosis (B20.0) according to the *International Classification of Diseases, tenth revision*. Geneva, World Health Organization, 1992. They are already counted in the number of deaths from HIV/AIDS (B20–B24). Source: *Global tuberculosis control: surveillance, planning, financing. WHO report 2007*. Geneva, World Health Organization, 2007 (WHO/HTM/TB/2007.376) (http://www.who.int/tb/publications/global_report).

Cause-specific mortality rate (per 100 000 population)			Age-standardized mortality rate by cause[h,i] (per 100 000 population)				Distribution of YLL by broader causes[h,j,k] (%)			Distribution of causes of death among children aged < 5 years[k,m] (%)							
HIV/AIDS[e]	TB among HIV-negative people[f]	TB among HIV-positive people[g]	Non-communicable diseases	Cardio-vascular diseases	Cancer	Injuries	Communicable diseases[l]	Non-communicable diseases	Injuries	Neonatal diseases	HIV/AIDS	Diarrhoeal diseases	Measles	Malaria	Pneumonia	Injuries	Other
Both sexes			Both sexes				Both sexes			Both sexes							
2005	2005	2005	2002	2002	2002	2002	2002	2002	2002	2000	2000	2000	2000	2000	2000	2000	2000
47	13	1	891	637	139	135	9	71	20	42.3	4.9	1.2	0.0	0.0	6.3	14.5	30.7
...	2	...	625	369	100	72	12	59	28	55.7	0.1	6.3	0.0	0.0	4.7	15.0	18.2
<10	1	<1	434	182	143	26	10	82	9	59.1	0.0	0.9	0.0	0.0	2.2	4.4	33.4
365	50	25	847	435	151	115	85	8	6	26.9	9.3	16.8	1.3	22.7	21.1	2.0	0.0
5	<1	<1	460	188	134	47	9	75	17	56.9	0.1	0.1	0.0	0.0	1.3	10.3	31.3
<50	3	<1	518	208	170	55	12	72	15	48.1	0.2	2.3	0.0	0.0	5.4	7.0	36.9
<10	15	<1	899	663	74	50	30	57	13	38.1	0.0	14.8	0.1	0.8	16.8	7.0	22.4
...	10	...	772	409	92	38	39	51	9	42.3	0.3	11.5	0.3	0.6	13.0	2.7	29.4
23	5	<1	496	241	107	90	24	45	32	52.6	0.2	9.9	0.0	0.0	5.9	6.5	24.8
15	22	<1	664	318	123	72	40	44	16	56.4	1.0	10.4	3.4	0.4	11.5	4.9	11.9
...	10	<1	956	553	108	102	61	28	11	33.3	0.3	16.1	2.2	7.5	19.8	3.7	17.1
840	60	57	700	359	122	58	92	6	2	22.9	16.1	17.5	1.2	19.4	21.8	1.0	0.1
1 384	61	69	685	347	122	103	90	7	4	28.1	40.6	12.1	2.9	0.2	14.7	1.2	0.3
<10	...	...	767	508	149	36	7	85	8	57.1	0.1	6.0	0.1	0.0	9.1	2.9	24.7
265	52	22	800	404	144	133	83	10	7	26.2	6.8	16.6	4.3	17.5	21.1	1.9	5.6
12	5	0	515	214	132	63	27	54	19	43.7	1.4	10.1	0.1	0.4	11.6	4.9	27.9
11	30	1	719	395	111	106	55	31	13	44.4	0.6	20.1	3.5	1.1	18.1	2.3	9.9
8	7	0	613	354	144	80	11	71	18	44.3	0.2	10.2	0.1	0.5	13.1	6.2	25.4
21	20	1	785	455	100	95	60	29	12	43.4	0.4	14.6	3.0	2.9	19.0	3.2	13.5
4	17	0	571	245	142	72	26	55	19	47.0	0.3	12.0	0.8	0.4	13.8	7.3	18.4
42	21	3	624	315	132	87	54	33	13	37	3	17	3	8	19	3	11

[h] *Mortality and burden of disease estimates for WHO Member States in 2002.* World Health Organization, December 2004 (http://www.who.int/entity/healthinfo/statistics/bodgbddeathdalyestimates.xls).

[i] Rates are age-standardized to WHO's world standard population. Source: Ahmad OB et al. *Age standardization of rates: a new WHO standard.* Geneva, World Health Organization, 2001 (GPE Discussion Paper Series No.31) (http://www.who.int/entity/healthinfo/paper31.pdf).

[j] YLL, years of life lost.

[k] The sum of individual proportions may not add up to 100% due to rounding.

[l] Communicable diseases include maternal causes, conditions arising during the perinatal period and nutritional deficiencies.

[m] Neonatal causes include diarrhoea occurring during the neonatal period. Sources: Bryce J et al. *WHO estimates of the causes of death in children. Lancet,* 2005, 365:1147–1152; Mortality profiles. Geneva, World Health Organization, 2007 (http://www.who.int/whosis/mort/profiles).

[n] Estimate will be finalized following completion of an ongoing analysis (as of March 2007) designed to reconcile results from multiple recent surveys.

[o] On 3 June 2006, the Permanent Representative of the Republic of Serbia to the United Nations and other International Organizations in Geneva informed the Acting Director-General of the WHO that *"the membership of the state union Serbia and Montenegro in the United Nations, including all organs and the organizations of the United Nations system, is continued by the Republic of Serbia on the basis of Article 60 of the Constitutional Charter of Serbia and Montenegro, activated by the Declaration of Independence adopted by the National Assembly of Montenegro on 3 June 2006".* Certain data, statistics and other factual elements used or referred to in this report cover a period of time preceding that communication. Consequently, the expression "Serbia and Montenegro" may appear with reference to the status of the Member State in question before the aforementioned communication. The use of that expression is without prejudice to the status of either the Republic of Serbia or of Montenegro in the light of the afore mentioned communication.

Health status: morbidity

Figures have been computed by WHO to ensure comparability; thus they are not necessarily the official statistics of Member States, which may use alternative rigorous methods.

	Member State	WHO region	HIV prevalence among adults aged ≥ 15 years[a] (per 100 000 population)	TB prevalence[b] (per 100 000 population)	TB incidence[b] (per 100 000 population)	No. confirmed cases of poliomyelitis[c]
			2005	2005	2005	2006
1	Afghanistan	EMR	<100	288	168	32
2	Albania	EUR	...	28	20	0
3	Algeria	AFR	82	55	55	0
4	Andorra	EUR	...	15	18	0
5	Angola	AFR	3 281	333	269	2
6	Antigua and Barbuda	AMR	...	9	7	0
7	Argentina	AMR	456	51	41	0
8	Armenia	EUR	121	79	71	0
9	Australia	WPR	99	6	6	0
10	Austria	EUR	173	9	11	0
11	Azerbaijan	EUR	87	85	76	0
12	Bahamas	AMR	2 807	49	38	0
13	Bahrain	EMR	...	43	40	0
14	Bangladesh	SEAR	<100	406	227	17
15	Barbados	AMR	1 236	12	11	0
16	Belarus	EUR	242	70	62	0
17	Belgium	EUR	162	10	13	0
18	Belize	AMR	2 110	55	49	0
19	Benin	AFR	1 635	144	88	0
20	Bhutan	SEAR	<100	174	103	0
21	Bolivia	AMR	120	280	211	0
22	Bosnia and Herzegovina	EUR	...	57	52	0
23	Botswana	AFR	23 624	556	654	0
24	Brazil	AMR	454	76	60	0
25	Brunei Darussalam	WPR	<100	63	54	0
26	Bulgaria	EUR	...	41	39	0
27	Burkina Faso	AFR	2 004	461	223	0
28	Burundi	AFR	3 132	602	334	0
29	Cambodia	WPR	1 468	703	506	1[d]
30	Cameroon	AFR	4 899	206	174	2
31	Canada	AMR	222	4	5	0
32	Cape Verde	AFR	...	327	174	0
33	Central African Republic	AFR	9 990	483	314	0
34	Chad	AFR	3 111	495	272	1
35	Chile	AMR	229	16	15	0
36	China	WPR	62	208	100	0
37	Colombia	AMR	509	66	45	0
38	Comoros	AFR	<500	89	45	0
39	Congo	AFR	4 731	449	367	0
40	Cook Islands	WPR	...	26	16	0
41	Costa Rica	AMR	235	17	14	0
42	Côte d'Ivoire	AFR	6 442	659	382	0
43	Croatia	EUR	...	65	41	0
44	Cuba	AMR	52	11	9	0
45	Cyprus	EUR	...	5	4	0
46	Czech Republic	EUR	<100	11	10	0
47	Democratic People's Republic of Korea	SEAR	...	179	178	0
48	Democratic Republic of the Congo	AFR	2 933	541	356	12
49	Denmark	EUR	125	6	7	0
50	Djibouti	EMR	3 017	1 161	762	0
51	Dominica	AMR	...	24	16	0
52	Dominican Republic	AMR	1 036	116	91	0
53	Ecuador	AMR	246	202	131	0
54	Egypt	EMR	<100	32	25	0
55	El Salvador	AMR	770	68	51	0

WORLD HEALTH STATISTICS 2007

	Member State	WHO region	HIV prevalence among adults aged ≥ 15 years[a] (per 100 000 population)	TB prevalence[b] (per 100 000 population)	TB incidence[b] (per 100 000 population)	No. confirmed cases of poliomyelitis[c]
			2005	2005	2005	2006
56	Equatorial Guinea	AFR	2 857	355	233	0
57	Eritrea	AFR	2 180	515	282	0
58	Estonia	EUR	887	46	43	0
59	Ethiopia	AFR	...	546	344	17
60	Fiji	WPR	<500	30	23	0
61	Finland	EUR	<100	5	6	0
62	France	EUR	263	10	13	0
63	Gabon	AFR	6 750	385	308	0
64	Gambia	AFR	2 091	352	242	0
65	Georgia	EUR	154	86	83	0
66	Germany	EUR	69	6	7	0
67	Ghana	AFR	2 225	380	205	0
68	Greece	EUR	98	15	17	0
69	Grenada	AMR	...	8	5	0
70	Guatemala	AMR	825	110	78	0
71	Guinea	AFR	1 475	431	236	0
72	Guinea-Bissau	AFR	3 483	293	206	0
73	Guyana	AMR	2 072	194	149	0
74	Haiti	AMR	3 377	405	305	0
75	Honduras	AMR	1 392	99	78	0
76	Hungary	EUR	<100	25	22	0
77	Iceland	EUR	<500	2	3	0
78	India	SEAR	747	299	168	660
79	Indonesia	SEAR	106	262	239	2
80	Iran (Islamic Republic of)	EMR	133	30	23	0
81	Iraq	EMR	...	76	56	0
82	Ireland	EUR	151	10	12	0
83	Israel	EUR	...	6	8	0
84	Italy	EUR	300	5	7	0
85	Jamaica	AMR	1 371	10	7	0
86	Japan	WPR	<100	38	28	0
87	Jordan	EMR	...	6	5	0
88	Kazakhstan	EUR	105	155	144	0
89	Kenya	AFR	6 125	936	641	2
90	Kiribati	WPR	...	426	380	0
91	Kuwait	EMR	...	28	24	0
92	Kyrgyzstan	EUR	111	133	121	0
93	Lao People's Democratic Republic	WPR	103	306	155	0
94	Latvia	EUR	508	66	63	0
95	Lebanon	EMR	114	12	11	0
96	Lesotho	AFR	22 684	588	696	0
97	Liberia	AFR	...	507	301	0
98	Libyan Arab Jamahiriya	EMR	...	18	18	0
99	Lithuania	EUR	116	63	63	0
100	Luxembourg	EUR	<500	9	11	0
101	Madagascar	AFR	451	396	234	0
102	Malawi	AFR	12 528	518	409	0
103	Malaysia	WPR	391	131	102	0
104	Maldives	SEAR	...	53	47	0
105	Mali	AFR	1 572	578	278	0
106	Malta	EUR	<500	4	6	0
107	Marshall Islands	WPR	...	269	224	0
108	Mauritania	AFR	629	590	298	0
109	Mauritius	AFR	437	132	62	0
110	Mexico	AMR	244	27	23	0

Health status: morbidity

Figures have been computed by WHO to ensure comparability; thus they are not necessarily the official statistics of Member States, which may use alternative rigorous methods.

	Member State	WHO region	HIV prevalence among adults aged ≥ 15 years[a] (per 100 000 population)	TB prevalence[b] (per 100 000 population)	TB incidence[b] (per 100 000 population)	No. confirmed cases of poliomyelitis[c]
			2005	2005	2005	2006
111	Micronesia (Federated States of)	WPR	...	123	105	0
112	Monaco	EUR	...	2	2	0
113	Mongolia	WPR	<100	206	191	0
114	Montenegro	EUR	...	42	33	0
115	Morocco	EMR	88	73	89	0
116	Mozambique	AFR	14 429	597	447	0
117	Myanmar	SEAR	982	170	171	1[d]
118	Namibia	AFR	17 676	577	697	19
119	Nauru	WPR	...	156	108	0
120	Nepal	SEAR	447	244	180	4
121	Netherlands	EUR	127	5	7	0
122	New Zealand	WPR	<100	9	9	0
123	Nicaragua	AMR	215	74	58	0
124	Niger	AFR	998	294	164	11
125	Nigeria	AFR	3 547	536	283	1 099[e]
126	Niue	WPR	...	87	44	0
127	Norway	EUR	67	4	5	0
128	Oman	EMR	...	11	11	0
129	Pakistan	EMR	86	297	181	40
130	Palau	WPR	...	61	52	0
131	Panama	AMR	755	46	45	0
132	Papua New Guinea	WPR	1 621	475	250	0
133	Paraguay	AMR	338	100	68	0
134	Peru	AMR	480	206	172	0
135	Philippines	WPR	<100	450	291	0
136	Poland	EUR	78	29	26	0
137	Portugal	EUR	363	25	33	0
138	Qatar	EMR	...	65	55	0
139	Republic of Korea	WPR	<100	135	96	0
140	Republic of Moldova	EUR	815	149	138	0
141	Romania	EUR	...	146	134	0
142	Russian Federation	EUR	775	150	119	0
143	Rwanda	AFR	3 133	673	361	0
144	Saint Kitts and Nevis	AMR	...	17	11	0
145	Saint Lucia	AMR	...	22	17	0
146	Saint Vincent and the Grenadines	AMR	...	42	29	0
147	Samoa	WPR	...	27	20	0
148	San Marino	EUR	...	5	6	0
149	Sao Tome and Principe	AFR	...	258	105	0
150	Saudi Arabia	EMR	...	58	41	0
151	Senegal	AFR	837	466	255	0
152	Serbia	EUR	...	42	33	0
153	Seychelles	AFR	...	56	34	0
154	Sierra Leone	AFR	1 361	905	475	0
155	Singapore	WPR	158	28	29	0
156	Slovakia	EUR	<100	20	17	0
157	Slovenia	EUR	<100	15	15	0
158	Solomon Islands	WPR	...	201	142	0
159	Somalia	EMR	870	286	224	36
160	South Africa	AFR	16 579	511	600	0
161	Spain	EUR	380	22	27	0
162	Sri Lanka	SEAR	<100	80	60	0
163	Sudan	EMR	1 454	400	228	0
164	Suriname	AMR	1 623	99	65	0
165	Swaziland	AFR	34 457	1 211	1 262	0

WORLD HEALTH STATISTICS 2007

	Member State	WHO region	HIV prevalence among adults aged ≥ 15 years[a] (per 100 000 population)	TB prevalence[b] (per 100 000 population)	TB incidence[b] (per 100 000 population)	No. confirmed cases of poliomyelitis[c]
			2005	2005	2005	2006
166	Sweden	EUR	107	5	6	0
167	Switzerland	EUR	264	6	7	0
168	Syrian Arab Republic	EMR	...	46	37	0
169	Tajikistan	EUR	123	297	198	0
170	Thailand	SEAR	1 144	204	142	0
171	The former Yugoslav Republic of Macedonia	EUR	<100	33	30	0
172	Timor-Leste	SEAR	...	713	556	0
173	Togo	AFR	2 879	753	373	0
174	Tonga	WPR	...	32	25	0
175	Trinidad and Tobago	AMR	2 538	13	9	0
176	Tunisia	EMR	115	28	24	0
177	Turkey	EUR	...	44	29	0
178	Turkmenistan	EUR	<100	90	70	0
179	Tuvalu	WPR	...	495	305	0
180	Uganda	AFR	6 304	559	369	0
181	Ukraine	EUR	1 036	120	99	0
182	United Arab Emirates	EMR	...	24	16	0
183	United Kingdom	EUR	137	11	14	0
184	United Republic of Tanzania	AFR	5 909	496	342	0
185	United States of America	AMR	508	3	5	0
186	Uruguay	AMR	362	33	28	0
187	Uzbekistan	EUR	174	139	113	0
188	Vanuatu	WPR	...	84	60	0
189	Venezuela (Bolivarian Republic of)	AMR	598	52	42	0
190	Viet Nam	WPR	421	235	175	0
191	Yemen	EMR	...	136	82	1
192	Zambia	AFR	15 819	618	600	0
193	Zimbabwe	AFR	19 210	631	601	0
194	The former state union of Serbia and Montenegro[f]	EUR	117	42	33	...

Region					
African Region	AFR	5 736	511	343	1 165
Region of the Americas	AMR	481	50	39	0
South-East Asia Region	SEAR	605	290	181	684
European Region	EUR	347	60	50	0
Eastern Mediterranean Region	EMR	207	163	104	109
Western Pacific Region	WPR	90	206	110	1
Global		803	217	136	1 959

... Data not available or not applicable; AFR, African Region; AMR, Region of the Americas; SEAR, South-East Asia Region; EUR, European Region; EMR, Eastern Mediterranean Region; WPR, Western Pacific Region.

The global values for rates and ratios are weighted averages; for absolute numbers they are the sums of all WHO regions.

[a] *2006 report on the global AIDS epidemic.* Geneva, Joint United Nations Programme on HIV/AIDS, World Health Organization, 2006. See Annex 2: HIV and AIDS estimates and data, 2005 and 2003. Ranges of estimates and notes are available from this document.

[b] TB, tuberculosis. Data are for all forms of TB including TB in people with HIV infection. Source: *Global tuberculosis control: surveillance, planning, financing. WHO report 2007*. Geneva, World Health Organization, 2007 (WHO/HTM/TB/2007.376) (http://www.who.int/tb/publications/global_report).

[c] Data from World Health Organization, Polio Eradication Initiative, as of 2 February 2007. Updated information can be found at http://www.who.int/immunization_monitoring/en/diseases/poliomyelitis/case_count.cfm.

[d] One case of vaccine-derived poliovirus infection.

[e] Of the total confirmed cases of poliomyelitis, one is vaccine-derived poliovirus.

[f] See footnote o to the table on Health status: mortality.

Health service coverage

Figures have been computed by WHO to ensure comparability; thus they are not necessarily the official statistics of Member States, which may use alternative rigorous methods.

	Member State	WHO region	Immunization coverage among 1-year-olds[a]			Antenatal care coverage[b]			Births attended by skilled health personnel[c]		Contraceptive prevalence rate[d]	
			Measles	DTP3	HepB3	At least 1 visit	At least 4 visits	Year				
			(%) 2005	(%) 2005	(%) 2005	(%)	(%)		(%)	Year	(%)	Year
1	Afghanistan	EMR	64	76	...	52	...	2003	14	2003	4.8	2000
2	Albania	EUR	97	98	98	81	42	2002	94	2002[k]	75.1	2002
3	Algeria	AFR	83	88	83	79	...	2000	90	2002	64.0	2000
4	Andorra	EUR	94	98	79	...	...		...		...	
5	Angola	AFR	45	47	...	...	...		45	2001	6.2	2001
6	Antigua and Barbuda	AMR	99	99	99	...	82	2001	100	2005	...	
7	Argentina	AMR	99	92	87	...	95	2001	99	2004[k]	...	
8	Armenia	EUR	94	90	91	82	65	2000	98	2005	60.5	2000
9	Australia	WPR	94	92	94	...	...		100	2003	...	
10	Austria	EUR	75	86	86	...	...		...		...	
11	Azerbaijan	EUR	98	93	96	70	...	2001	74	2001	55.4	2001
12	Bahamas	AMR	85	93	93	...	...		99	2004	...	
13	Bahrain	EMR	99	98	98	...	...		99	2005	...	
14	Bangladesh	SEAR	81	88	62	39	11	1999–2000	13	2004[k]	58.1	2004
15	Barbados	AMR	93	92	92	89	...	2001	100	2004	...	
16	Belarus	EUR	99	99	99	...	...		100	2005	...	
17	Belgium	EUR	88	97	78	...	...		99	1999	...	
18	Belize	AMR	95	96	97	...	96	2001	89	2005	...	
19	Benin	AFR	85	93	92	88	61	2001	66	2001[k]	18.6	2001
20	Bhutan	SEAR	93	95	95	...	...		51	2005	...	
21	Bolivia	AMR	64	81	81	84	69	2001	61	2003–2004[k]	58.4	2003–2004
22	Bosnia and Herzegovina	EUR	90	93	93	99	...	2000	100	2000	47.5	2000
23	Botswana	AFR	90	97	85	99	97	2001	99	2000	40.4	2000
24	Brazil	AMR	99	96	92	...	...		97	2003	...	
25	Brunei Darussalam	WPR	97	99	99	...	100	2001	100	2004	...	
26	Bulgaria	EUR	96	96	96	...	...		99	2005	41.5	1997
27	Burkina Faso	AFR	84	96	...	72	18	2003	38	2003	13.8	2003
28	Burundi	AFR	75	74	74	93	79	2001	25	2000	15.7	2000
29	Cambodia	WPR	79	82	...	44	9	2000	44	2005–2006	23.8	2000
30	Cameroon	AFR	68	80	79	77	52	1998	62	2004	26.0	2004
31	Canada	AMR	94	94	...	...	...		100	2003–2004	...	
32	Cape Verde	AFR	65	73	69	...	99	2001	89	1998[k]	52.9	1998
33	Central African Republic	AFR	35	40	...	...	...		44	2000	27.9	2000
34	Chad	AFR	23	20	...	51	13	1997	15	2004–2005[k]	2.8	2004
35	Chile	AMR	90	91	...	...	...		100	2004	...	
36	China	WPR	86	87	84	...	...		83	2004	90.2	2004
37	Colombia	AMR	89	87	87	90	79	2000	91	2004–2005	78.2	2004–2005
38	Comoros	AFR	80	80	80	...	...		62	2000	25.7	2000
39	Congo	AFR	56	65	...	...	...		83	2005–2006[k]	44.3	2005
40	Cook Islands	WPR	99	99	99	...	...		98	2001	...	
41	Costa Rica	AMR	89	91	90	...	70	2001	98	2004	80.0	1999
42	Côte d'Ivoire	AFR	51	56	56	84	35	1998–1999	63	2000	15.0	1998–1999
43	Croatia	EUR	96	96	99	...	...		100	2005	...	
44	Cuba	AMR	98	99	99	...	100	2001	100	2005	73.3	2000
45	Cyprus	EUR	86	98	88	...	...		99	2003	...	

WORLD HEALTH STATISTICS 2007

Children aged <5 years sleeping under insecticide-treated bednets[e]		Antiretroviral therapy coverage		TB detection rate under DOTS[h]	TB treatment success under DOTS[i]	Children aged < 5 years with ARI symptoms taken to facility[j]		Children aged < 5 years with diarrhoea receiving ORT[j]		Children aged < 5 years with fever who received treatment with any antimalarial[e]		Children 6–59 months who received vitamin A supplementation[j]		Births by Caesarean section[b]	
		People with advanced HIV infections[f]	HIV-infected pregnant women for PMTCT[g]												
(%)	Year	(%) Dec 2006	(%) Dec 2005	(%) 2005	(%) 2004 cohort	(%)	Year	(%)	Year	(%)	Year	(%)	Year	(%)	Year
...		...	...	44	89	...		...		...		...		...	
...		...	...	25	78	...		...		...		...		15	2002
...		25	...	106	91	...		...		...		...		6	2000
...		...	...	94	100	...		...		...		...		24	1999
2	2001	10	1	85	68					63.0	2001	...		...	
...		...	...	246	100	...		...		...		...		...	
...		79	87	67	58	...		...		...		...		...	
...		...	...	60	70	24.6	2000	59.7	2000	...		...		7	2000
...		...	...	42	85	...		...		...		...		21	1998
...		...	...	56	69	...		...		...		...		21	2002
1	2000	<1	...	55	60	...		...		0.8	2000	...		4	2002
...		...	...	...	...	...		...		...		...		...	
...		...	...	77	82	...		...		...		...		...	
...		<3	...	59	90	20.3	2004	83.4	2004	...		81.8	2004	3	1999–2000
...		87	...	...	...	...		...		...		...		...	
...		20	...	46	74	...		...		...		...		17	2002
...		...	...	64	72	...		...		...		...		16	1999
...		59	...	102	60	...		...		...		...		...	
7	2001	38	17	83	83	29.3	2001	60.9	2001	60.4	2001	...		4	2001
...		...	...	31	83	...		...		...		...		...	
...		24	...	72	80	51.5	2003	66.4	2003	...		60.0	2003	15	1998
...		...	...	71	98	...		...		...		...		...	
...		>95	54	69	65	...		...		...		...		...	
...		85	48	53	81	...		...		...		...		...	
...		...	...	112	71	...		...		...		...		...	
...		...	...	90	80	...		...		...		...		17	2002
2	2003	39	6	18	67	32.6	2003	62.8	2003	49.6	2003	33.3	2003	1	2003
1	2000	26	3	30	78	...		...		31.3	2000	...		...	
...		...	4	66	91	34.5	2000	74.1	2000	...		28.5	2000	1	2000
1	2004	25	10	106	71	39.9	2004	56.7	2004	53.1	2004	37.5	2004	3	1998
...		...	...	64	62	...		...		...		...		19	1997–1998
...		...	...	34	71	...		...		...		...		6	1998
2	2000	6	4	40	91	...		...		68.8	2000	...		...	
1	2000	14	1	22	69	11.8	2004	37.5	2004	55.8	2004	32.0	2004	1	1996–1997
...		83	...	112	83	...		...		...		...		...	
...		27	2	80	94	...		...		...		...		...	
3	2000	50	...	26	85	56.7	2005	70.1	2005	...		...		25	2000
9	2000	...	...	49	94	...		...		62.7	2000	...		...	
...		17	10	57	63	43.9	2005	53.5	2005	...		65.5	2005	...	
...		...	...	77	0	...		...		...		...		...	
...		>95	...	118	...	...		...		...		...		...	
1	2000	28	4	38	71	34.9	1999	66.1	1999	57.5	2000	...		3	1998–1999
...		...	...	...	...	...		...		...		...		14	2002
...		>95	...	98	93	...		...		...		...		...	
...		...	...	57	20	...		...		...		...		...	

Health service coverage

Figures have been computed by WHO to ensure comparability; thus they are not necessarily the official statistics of Member States, which may use alternative rigorous methods.

	Member State	WHO region	Immunization coverage among 1-year-olds[a]			Antenatal care coverage[b]			Births attended by skilled health personnel[c]		Contraceptive prevalence rate[d]	
			Measles	DTP3	HepB3	At least 1 visit	At least 4 visits	Year				
			(%) 2005	(%) 2005	(%) 2005	(%)	(%)		(%)	Year	(%)	Year
46	Czech Republic	EUR	97	97	99	...	...		100	2005	72.0	1997
47	Democratic People's Republic of Korea	SEAR	96	79	92	98	...	2000	97	2004	...	
48	Democratic Republic of the Congo	AFR	70	73	...	...	...		61	2001	31.4	2001
49	Denmark	EUR	95	93	...	...	...		...		...	
50	Djibouti	EMR	65	71	...	...	...		61	2003	...	
51	Dominica	AMR	98	98	...	...	100	2001	100	2004	...	
52	Dominican Republic	AMR	99	77	77	100	93	1999	98	2002[k]	69.8	2002
53	Ecuador	AMR	93	94	94	56	...	1999	74	2004	65.8	1999
54	Egypt	EMR	98	98	98	54	41	2000	74	2005	59.2	2005
55	El Salvador	AMR	99	89	89	...	76	2001	69	2002–2003	67.3	2002–2003
56	Equatorial Guinea	AFR	51	33	...	...	37	2001	65	2000	...	
57	Eritrea	AFR	84	83	83	...	49	2001	28	2002	8.0	2002
58	Estonia	EUR	96	96	95	...	...		100	2005	...	
59	Ethiopia	AFR	59	69	...	27	10	2000	6	2005	14.7	2005
60	Fiji	WPR	70	75	75	...	...		99	2002	...	
61	Finland	EUR	97	97	...	...	...		100	2002	...	
62	France	EUR	87	98	29	...	...		...		...	
63	Gabon	AFR	55	38	55	94	63	2000	86	2000[k]	32.7	2000
64	Gambia	AFR	84	88	88	92	...	2000	55	2000	9.6	2000
65	Georgia	EUR	92	84	74	91	...	1999	92	2005	47.2	2005
66	Germany	EUR	93	90	84	...	...		100	2006	...	
67	Ghana	AFR	83	84	84	90	69	2003	47	2003	25.2	2003
68	Greece	EUR	88	88	88	...	...		...		...	
69	Grenada	AMR	99	99	99	...	98	2001	100	2005	...	
70	Guatemala	AMR	77	81	27	86	68	1998–1999	41	2002[k]	43.3	2002
71	Guinea	AFR	59	69	...	74	48	1999	38	2005	9.1	2005
72	Guinea-Bissau	AFR	80	80	...	89	62	2001	35	2000	7.6	2000
73	Guyana	AMR	92	93	93	88	...	2000	86	2000[k]	37.3	2000
74	Haiti	AMR	54	43	...	79	42	2000	25	2005–2006	28.1	2000
75	Honduras	AMR	92	91	91	...	84	2001	67	2005–2006	61.8	2001
76	Hungary	EUR	99	99	...	...	...		100	2005	...	
77	Iceland	EUR	90	95	...	...	...		...		...	
78	India	SEAR	58	59	8	65	30	1998–1999	48	2005–2006[k]	48.2	1998–1999
79	Indonesia	SEAR	72	70	70	97	81	2002–2003	66	2002–2003	60.3	2002–2003
80	Iran (Islamic Republic of)	EMR	94	95	94	...	77	2001	90	2000	72.9	1997
81	Iraq	EMR	90	81	81	...	78	2001	72	2000	...	
82	Ireland	EUR	84	90	...	...	...		100	2002	...	
83	Israel	EUR	95	95	95	...	...		...		...	
84	Italy	EUR	87	96	96	...	...		99	2003	...	
85	Jamaica	AMR	84	88	87	...	99	2001	97	2002–2003	65.9	1997
86	Japan	WPR	99	99	...	...	...		100	2004	55.9	2000
87	Jordan	EMR	95	95	95	99	91	2002	100	2002	55.8	2002
88	Kazakhstan	EUR	99	98	94	82	71	1999	99	2005	66.1	1999
89	Kenya	AFR	69	76	76	88	52	2003	42	2003	39.3	2003
90	Kiribati	WPR	56	62	67	...	88	2001	89	2002	...	

World Health Statistics 2007

Children aged <5 years sleeping under insecticide-treated bednets[a]		Antiretroviral therapy coverage		TB detection rate under DOTS[h]	TB treatment success under DOTS[i]	Children aged < 5 years with ARI symptoms taken to facility[j]		Children aged < 5 years with diarrhoea receiving ORT[l]		Children aged < 5 years with fever who received treatment with any antimalarial[n]		Children 6–59 months who received vitamin A supplementation[j]		Births by Caesarean section[u]	
		People with advanced HIV infections[t]	HIV-infected pregnant women for PMTCT[b]												
(%)	Year	(%) Dec 2006	(%) Dec 2005	(%) 2005	(%) 2004 cohort	(%)	Year	(%)	Year	(%)	Year	(%)	Year	(%)	Year
...		...	...	65	73	...		...		...		...		14	2002
...		...	...	99	89	...		...		...		...		...	
1	2001	11	2	72	85	...		...		45.4	2001	...		...	
...		...	...	71	88	...		...		...		...		18	2001
...		20	1	42	80	...		...		...		...		...	
...		...	...	...	...	...		...		...		...		...	
...		37	27	76	80	60.8	2002	55.0	2002	...		30.7	2002	32	1999
...		34	22	28	85	...		...		...		...		19	1999
...		22	...	63	70	72.6	2005	35.7	2005	...		13.8	2005	11	2000
...		39	18	67	90	...		...		...		...		16	1998
1	2000	24	...	...	...	...		...		48.6	2000	...		...	
4	2002	8	2	13	85	43.6	2002	68.4	2002	3.6	2002	38.0	2002	...	
...		...	...	64	71	...		...		...		...		15	2002
...		...	...	33	79	18.7	2005	37.1	2005	3.0	2000	45.8	2005	1	2000
...		...	...	72	...	...		...		...		...		...	
...		...	...	...	...	...		...		...		...		16	2002
...		...	...	...	...	...		...		...		...		16	1999
...		35	3	57	40	47.7	2000	71.6	2000	...		...		6	2000
15	2000	12	6	69	86	...		...		55.2	2000	...		...	
...		32	...	91	68	...		...		...		...		12	2002
...		...	...	52	68	...		...		...		...		22	2001
4	2003	16	6	37	72	44.0	2003	63.3	2003	62.8	2003	78.4	2003	4	2003
...		...	...	...	...	...		...		...		...		...	
...		...	...	...	...	...		...		...		...		...	
1	2000	52	10	55	85	37.4	1999	58.6	1999	...		...		12	1998–1999
...		10	1	56	72	34.5	2005	56.7	2005	...		68.2	2005	2	1999
7	2000	6	...	79	75	...		...		58.4	2000	...		...	
...		72	...	40	72	...		...		2.6	2000	...		...	
...		39	7	57	80	36.3	2000	54.9	2000	11.7	2000	31.6	2000	2	2000
...		40	12	82	85	55.9	2005	66.8	2005	...		...		...	
...		...	...	43	54	...		...		...		...		23	2002
...		...	...	53	50	...		...		...		...		17	2001
...		...	2	61	86	...		...		...		...		7	1998–1999
0	2000	20	<1	66	90	56.8	2003	60.6	2003	0.7	2002–2003	75.1	2003	4	2002–2003
...		5	...	64	84	...		...		...		...		...	
<0.1	2000	0	...	43	85	...		...		...		...		...	
...		...	...	...	...	...		...		...		...		19	2000
...		...	...	42	80	...		...		...		...		17	2001
...		...	...	72	...	...		...		...		...		32	1999
...		56	...	61	46	...		...		...		...		...	
...		...	...	57	57	...		...		...		...		...	
...		...	...	63	85	71.7	2002	63.9	2002	...		...		16	2002
...		10	...	72	72	48.0	1999	52.6	1999	...		...		11	1998
5	2003	44	20	43	80	45.5	2003	50.6	2003	26.5	2003	33.3	2003	4	2003
...		...	...	73	94	...		...		...		...		...	

Health service coverage

Figures have been computed by WHO to ensure comparability; thus they are not necessarily the official statistics of Member States, which may use alternative rigorous methods.

	Member State	WHO region	Immunization coverage among 1-year-olds[a]			Antenatal care coverage[b]			Births attended by skilled health personnel[c]		Contraceptive prevalence rate[d]	
			Measles	DTP3	HepB3	At least 1 visit	At least 4 visits	Year				
			(%) 2005	(%) 2005	(%) 2005	(%)	(%)		(%)	Year	(%)	Year
91	Kuwait	EMR	99	99	99	...	...		100	2002	...	
92	Kyrgyzstan	EUR	99	98	97	88	81	1997	98	2005	59.5	1997
93	Lao People's Democratic Republic	WPR	41	49	49	44	29	2001	19	2001	32.2	2000
94	Latvia	EUR	95	99	98	...	...		100	2005	...	
95	Lebanon	EMR	96	92	88	...	87	2001	98	2004	...	
96	Lesotho	AFR	85	83	83	91	88	2001	55	2004[k]	37.3	2004
97	Liberia	AFR	94	87	...	...	84	2001	51	1999–2000	...	
98	Libyan Arab Jamahiriya	EMR	97	98	97	...	81	2001	99	1999	...	
99	Lithuania	EUR	97	94	95	...	...		100	2005	...	
100	Luxembourg	EUR	95	99	95	...	...		100	2002	...	
101	Madagascar	AFR	59	61	61	91	38	1997	51	2003–2004	27.1	2003–2004
102	Malawi	AFR	82	93	93	94	55	2000	56	2004–2005	32.5	2004
103	Malaysia	WPR	90	90	90	...	...		100	2005	...	
104	Maldives	SEAR	97	98	98	98	81	2001	70	2001[k]	42.0	1999
105	Mali	AFR	86	85	85	53	30	2001	41	2001	8.1	2001
106	Malta	EUR	86	92	78	...	...		100	2006	...	
107	Marshall Islands	WPR	86	77	89	...	...		95	2002	...	
108	Mauritania	AFR	61	71	42	63	16	2000–2001	57	2000–2001[k]	8.0	2000–2001
109	Mauritius	AFR	98	97	97	...	...		99	2005	75.9	2002
110	Mexico	AMR	96	98	98	...	86	2001	93	2003	68.4	1997
111	Micronesia (Federated States of)	WPR	96	94	91	...	...		88	2001	...	
112	Monaco	EUR	99	99	99	...	...		...		...	
113	Mongolia	WPR	99	99	98	...	97	2001	100	2004	67.4	2000
114	Montenegro	EUR	...	...	...	...	...		...		...	
115	Morocco	EMR	97	98	96	...	...		63	2003–2004	63.0	2003–2004
116	Mozambique	AFR	77	72	72	71	41	1997	48	2003–2004	16.5	2003–2004
117	Myanmar	SEAR	72	73	62	...	76	2001	68	2003	37.0	2001
118	Namibia	AFR	73	86	...	85	69	2000	76	2000	43.7	2000
119	Nauru	WPR	80	80	80	...	...		...		...	
120	Nepal	SEAR	74	75	41	49	15	2001	19	2006	39.3	2001
121	Netherlands	EUR	96	98	...	...	...		100	2003	...	
122	New Zealand	WPR	82	89	87	...	...		97	2001	...	
123	Nicaragua	AMR	96	86	86	85	72	2001	67	2001	68.6	2001
124	Niger	AFR	83	89	...	39	11	1998	16	2000[k]	14.0	2000
125	Nigeria	AFR	35	25	...	61	47	2003	35	2003[k]	12.6	2003
126	Niue	WPR	99	85	86	...	...		100	2005	...	
127	Norway	EUR	90	91	...	...	...		...		...	
128	Oman	EMR	98	99	99	...	...		98	2005	...	
129	Pakistan	EMR	78	72	73	...	...		31	2004–2005	27.6	2000–2001
130	Palau	WPR	98	98	98	...	...		100	2002	...	
131	Panama	AMR	99	85	85	...	72	2001	91	2004	...	
132	Papua New Guinea	WPR	60	61	63	...	78	2001	42	2004	...	
133	Paraguay	AMR	90	75	75	...	89	2001	77	2004	72.8	2004
134	Peru	AMR	80	84	84	85	69	2000	71	2004[k]	70.5	2003–2004
135	Philippines	WPR	80	79	44	94	70	2003	60	2003	48.9	2003

WORLD HEALTH STATISTICS 2007

Children aged <5 years sleeping under insecticide-treated bednets[a]		Antiretroviral therapy coverage		TB detection rate under DOTS[h]	TB treatment success under DOTS[i]	Children aged < 5 years with ARI symptoms taken to facility[j]		Children aged < 5 years with diarrhoea receiving ORT[f]		Children aged < 5 years with fever who received treatment with any antimalarial[e]		Children 6–59 months who received vitamin A supplementation[f]		Births by Caesarean section[b]	
		People with advanced HIV infections[c]	HIV-infected pregnant women for PMTCT[d]												
(%)	Year	(%) Dec 2006	(%) Dec 2005	(%) 2005	(%) 2004 cohort	(%)	Year	(%)	Year	(%)	Year	(%)	Year	(%)	Year
...		...	...	66	63	...		...		...		...		...	
...		...	...	67	85	...		73.5	1997	...		...		6	1997
15	2002	...	...	68	86	...		...		...		...		...	
...		...	...	83	73	...		...		...		...		17	2002
...	...	...	...	74	90	...		...		...		...		23	1998
		31	12	85	69	54.4	2005	79.6	2005	...		54.6	2005	...	
...		...	...	50	70	...		...		...		...		...	
...		...	...	178	64	...		...		...		...		...	
...		...	...	100	72	...		...		...		...		15	2002
...		...	...	59	...	...		...		...		...		19	2000
0	2000	1	<1	67	71	39.3	2004	58.1	2004	41.1	2004	76.2	2004	1	1997
36	2004	43	6	39	71	19.6	2004	70.1	2004	31.6	2004	65.4	2004	3	2000
...		22	10	73	56	...		...		...		...		...	
...		...	...	94	95	...		...		...		...		...	
...		37	3	21	71	42.8	2001	65.7	2001	37.6	2003	40.9	2001	1	2001
...		...	...	50	100	...		...		...		...		25	2002
...		...	...	77	90	...		...		...		...		...	
2	2003-2004	17	1	28	22	39.4	2001	47.7	2001	33.4	2003–2004	57.8	2001	3	2000–2001
...		...	...	32	89	...		...		...		...		...	
...		76	...	110	82	...		...		...		...		...	
...		...	...	61	80	...		...		...		...		...	
...		...	...	...	...	...		...		...		...		...	
...		...	...	82	88	...		...		...		...		5	2000
...		...	...	...	...	...		...		...		...		...	
...		41	...	101	87	34.5	2004	54.0	2004	...		25.5	2004	...	
...		14	6	49	77	51.4	2003	70.5	2003	...		49.8	2003	3	1997
...		7	8	95	84	...		...		...		...		...	
...		71	29	90	68	53.1	2000	65.8	2000	14.4	2000	38.1	2000	...	
...		...	...	...	...	...		...		...		...		...	
...		4	...	67	87	23.7	2001	46.5	2001	...		81.0	2001	1	2001
...		...	...	47	83	...		...		...		...		14	2002
...		...	...	51	66	...		...		...		...		19	1999
...		35	...	88	87	57.4	2001	67.7	2001	1.8	2001	65.3	2001	15	2001
1	2000	6	1	50	61	28.1	2006	52.9	2006	48.1	2000	...		1	1998
1	2003	15	<1	22	73	31.4	2003	40.2	2003	33.8	2003	33.7	2003	2	2003
...		...	...	0	0	...		...		...		...		...	
...		...	...	44	89	...		...		...		...		16	2001
...		...	...	108	90	...		...		...		...		...	
...		<1	...	37	82	...		...		...		...		...	
...		...	...	64	100	...		...		...		...		...	
...		70	...	131	78	...		...		...		...		...	
...		8	1	21	65	...		...		...		...		...	
...		64	...	33	83	...		...		...		...		...	
...		50	9	86	90	68.0	2004	70.6	2004	...		...		13	2000
...		10	...	75	87	46.3	2003	58.9	2003	...		76.0	2003	7	2003

Health service coverage

Figures have been computed by WHO to ensure comparability; thus they are not necessarily the official statistics of Member States, which may use alternative rigorous methods.

	Member State	WHO region	Immunization coverage among 1-year-olds[a]			Antenatal care coverage[b]			Births attended by skilled health personnel[c]		Contraceptive prevalence rate[d]	
			Measles	DTP3	HepB3	At least 1 visit	At least 4 visits	Year				
			(%) 2005	(%) 2005	(%) 2005	(%)	(%)		(%)	Year	(%)	Year
136	Poland	EUR	98	99	98	...	...		100	2005	...	
137	Portugal	EUR	93	93	94	...	...		100	2001	...	
138	Qatar	EMR	99	97	97	62	58	1998	100	2002	43.2	1998
139	Republic of Korea	WPR	99	96	99	...	...		100	2003	80.5	1997
140	Republic of Moldova	EUR	97	98	99	99	...	1997	100	2005[j]	62.4	2000
141	Romania	EUR	97	97	98	89	...	1999	98	2005	63.8	1999
142	Russian Federation	EUR	99	98	97	96	...	1999	99	2005	72.8	1999
143	Rwanda	AFR	89	95	95	93	10	2001	39	2005[k]	13.2	2000
144	Saint Kitts and Nevis	AMR	99	99	99	...	100	2001	100	2005	...	
145	Saint Lucia	AMR	94	95	95	...	100	2001	100	2004	...	
146	Saint Vincent and the Grenadines	AMR	97	99	99	...	92	2001	100	2005	...	
147	Samoa	WPR	57	64	60	...	...		100	2004	...	
148	San Marino	EUR	94	95	95	...	...		...		...	
149	Sao Tome and Principe	AFR	88	97	96	91	...	2000	79	2000	29.3	2000
150	Saudi Arabia	EMR	96	96	96	...	...		96	2004	...	
151	Senegal	AFR	74	84	84	82	64	1999	52	2005	11.8	2005
152	Serbia	EUR	96	98	65	...	...		...		...	
153	Seychelles	AFR	99	99	99	...	...		...		...	
154	Sierra Leone	AFR	67	64	...	82	68	2001	42	2000	4.3	2000
155	Singapore	WPR	96	96	96	...	...		100	2004	62.0	1997
156	Slovakia	EUR	98	99	99	...	...		100	2004	...	
157	Slovenia	EUR	94	96	...	...	...		100	2005	...	
158	Solomon Islands	WPR	72	80	72	...	...		85	1999	...	
159	Somalia	EMR	35	35	...	...	32	2001	25	2002	...	
160	South Africa	AFR	82	94	94	89	72	1998	92	2003–2004	56.3	1998
161	Spain	EUR	97	96	96	...	...		...		...	
162	Sri Lanka	SEAR	99	99	99	...	98	2001	97	2000	70.0	2000
163	Sudan	EMR	60	59	52	...	75	2001	57	1999[m]	...	
164	Suriname	AMR	91	83	83	91	91	2001	71	2000[k]	42.1	2000
165	Swaziland	AFR	60	71	71	...	...		70	2000	27.7	2000
166	Sweden	EUR	94	99	...	...	...		...		...	
167	Switzerland	EUR	82	93	...	...	...		100	2006	...	
168	Syrian Arab Republic	EMR	98	99	99	...	51	2001	90	2004	...	
169	Tajikistan	EUR	84	81	81	75	...	2000	71	2000	33.9	2000
170	Thailand	SEAR	96	98	96	...	86	2001	99	2000	72.2	1996–1997
171	The former Yugoslav Republic of Macedonia	EUR	96	97	53	...	...		99	2005	...	
172	Timor-Leste	SEAR	48	55	...	...	...		18	2002	10.0	2003
173	Togo	AFR	70	82	...	78	46	1998	49	2000	25.7	2000
174	Tonga	WPR	99	99	99	...	...		98	2004	...	
175	Trinidad and Tobago	AMR	93	95	95	96	98	2001	97	2002	38.2	2000
176	Tunisia	EMR	96	98	97	...	79	2001	90	2000	63.0	2001
177	Turkey	EUR	91	90	85	67	42	1998	83	2003	63.9	1998
178	Turkmenistan	EUR	99	99	99	87	83	2000	97	2000	61.8	2000
179	Tuvalu	WPR	62	93	79	...	...		100	2002	...	
180	Uganda	AFR	86	84	84	92	40	2000–2001	39	2000–2001	22.8	2000–2001

World Health Statistics 2007

Children aged <5 years sleeping under insecticide-treated bednets[e]		Antiretroviral therapy coverage		TB detection rate under DOTS[h]	TB treatment success under DOTS[i]	Children aged < 5 years with ARI symptoms taken to facility[j]		Children aged < 5 years with diarrhoea receiving ORT[j]		Children aged < 5 years with fever who received treatment with any antimalarial[o]		Children 6–59 months who received vitamin A supplementation[j]		Births by Caesarean section[h]	
		People with advanced HIV infections[f]	HIV-infected pregnant women for PMTCT[g]												
(%)	Year	(%) Dec 2006	(%) Dec 2005	(%) 2005	(%) 2004 cohort	(%)	Year	(%)	Year	(%)	Year	(%)	Year	(%)	Year
...	...	...	...	62	79	...		...		...		...		...	
...	...	...	...	85	84	...		...		...		...		30	2001
...	...	...	...	47	78	...		...		...		...		16	1998
...	...	...	...	18	80	...		...		...		...		...	
...	...	...	6	65	62	54.4	2005	...		...		...		6	1997
...	...	...	...	82	82	...		...		...		...		11	1999
...	...	11	84	30	59	...		...		...		...		12	1999
5	2000	72	36	29	77	26.9	2005	31.9	2005	12.6	2000	84.1	2005	2	2000
...		...	...	0	...	...		...		...		...		...	
...		...	...	92	64	...		...		...		...		...	
...		...	...	39	86	...		...		...		...		...	
...		...	...	66	100	...		...		...		...		...	
...		...	...	...	...	...		...		...		...		...	
23	2000	...	...	...	...	...		...		61.2	2000	...		...	
...		...	...	38	82	...		...		...		...		...	
2	2000	34	1	51	74	40.6	2005	52.5	2005	36.2	2000	75.3	2005	2	1997
...		...	...	79	91	...		...		...		...		...	
...		...	...	65	92	...		...		...		...		...	
2	2000	14	1	37	82	...		...		60.7	2000	...		2	1997
...		...	...	100	81	...		...		...		...		...	
...		...	...	39	88	...		...		...		...		18	2002
...		...	...	84	90	...		...		...		...		14	2002
...		...	...	55	87	...		...		...		...		...	
0	1999	<1	...	86	91	...		...		18.5	1999	...		...	
...		33	30	103	70	75.3	1998	89.1	1998	...		...		16	1998
...		...	...	...	...	...		...		...		...		...	
...		< 8	...	86	85	...		...		...		...		...	
0	2000	1	<1	35	77	...		...		50.2	2000	...		...	
3	2000	93	...	...	...	...		...		...		...		...	
0	2000	42	34	42	50	...		...		25.5	2000	...		...	
...		...	...	56	64	...		...		...		...		17	2001
...		...	...	...	...	...		...		...		...		10	2002
...		...	...	42	86	...		...		...		...		...	
2	2000	<5	12	22	84	...		...		68.9	2000	...		2	2002
...		88	...	73	74	...		...		...		...		...	
...		...	...	66	84	...		...		...		...		10	2001
4	2002	0	...	44	80	...		...		47.4	2002	...		...	
2	2000	24	8	18	67	...		...		60.0	2000	...		2	1998
...		...	...	96	...	...		...		...		...		...	
...		45	...	...	...	...		...		...		...		...	
...		...	...	82	90	...		...		...		...		8	2000
...		...	...	3	91	41.0	2003	...		...		...		14	1998
...		...	...	43	86	...		...		...		...		4	2000
...		...	...	35	100	...		...		...		...		...	
0	2000-2001	41	11	45	70	29.6	2001	53.1	2001	...		37.6	2001	3	2000–2001

Health service coverage

Figures have been computed by WHO to ensure comparability; thus they are not necessarily the official statistics of Member States, which may use alternative rigorous methods.

	Member State	WHO region	Immunization coverage among 1-year-olds[a]			Antenatal care coverage[b]			Births attended by skilled health personnel[c]		Contraceptive prevalence rate[d]	
			Measles	DTP3	HepB3	At least 1 visit	At least 4 visits	Year				
			(%) 2005	(%) 2005	(%) 2005	(%)	(%)		(%)	Year	(%)	Year
181	Ukraine	EUR	96	96	97	90	...	1999	100	2005	67.5	1999
182	United Arab Emirates	EMR	92	94	92	...	...		100	2003	...	
183	United Kingdom	EUR	82	91	...	...	...		99	1998	84.0	2002
184	United Republic of Tanzania	AFR	91	90	90	96	69	1999	46	2004–2005	26.4	2004–2005
185	United States of America	AMR	93	96	92	...	...		99	2003	72.9	2002
186	Uruguay	AMR	95	96	96	...	94	2001	99	2004	...	
187	Uzbekistan	EUR	99	99	99	...	...		96	2000	67.7	2002
188	Vanuatu	WPR	70	66	56	...	...		87	2003	...	
189	Venezuela (Bolivarian Republic of)	AMR	76	87	88	...	90	2001	94	2000	...	
190	Viet Nam	WPR	95	95	94	70	29	2002	85	2002	78.5	2002
191	Yemen	EMR	76	86	86	34	11	1997	20	2003	20.8	1997
192	Zambia	AFR	84	80	80	94	71	2001–2002	43	2001–2002	34.2	2001–2002
193	Zimbabwe	AFR	85	90	90	82	64	1999	80	2005–2006	53.5	1999
194	The former state union of Serbia and Montenegro[n]	EUR	...	...	...	...	...		93	2001	58.3	2000
Region												
	African Region	AFR	65	67	39	...	...		44		23.7	
	Region of the Americas	AMR	92	92	85	...	...		91		72.0	
	South-East Asia Region	SEAR	65	66	27	...	...		49		51.5	
	European Region	EUR	93	95	76	...	...		95		68.3	
	Eastern Mediterranean Region	EMR	82	82	74	...	...		53		39.9	
	Western Pacific Region	WPR	87	87	76	...	...		81		84.7	
	Global		77	78	55	...	...		63		61.9	

... Data not available or not applicable; AFR, African Region; AMR, Region of the Americas; SEAR, South-East Asia Region; EUR, European Region; EMR, Eastern Mediterranean Region; WPR, Western Pacific Region.

The global values for rates and ratios are weighted averages; for absolute numbers they are the sums of all WHO regions.

[a] DTP3, 3 doses of diphtheria–tetanus toxoid–pertussis vaccine; HepB3, 3 doses of Hepatitis B vaccine. *WHO/UNICEF estimates of national immunization coverage* [online database.]. Geneva, World Health Organization, 2006 (http://www.who.int/immunization_monitoring/routine/immunization_coverage/en/index4.html). Estimates based on data available up to August 2006. For countries recommending the first dose of measles among children older than 12 months of age, the indicator is calculated as the proportion of children less than 24 months of age receiving one dose of measles containing vaccine.

[b] *The World Health Report 2005: make every mother and child count.* Geneva, World Health Organization, 2005 (http://www.who.int/whr/2005/en/index.html).

[c] *WHO global database on births attended by skill health personnel*, Geneva, World Health Organization, 2007.

[d] Percentage of women using contraception among those of reproductive age who are married or living with a partner. Source: *World contraceptive use 2005* [CD-ROM]. New York, Population Division, Department of Economic and Social Affairs, United Nations Secretariat, 2006. Additional updated information obtained by WHO's Department of Reproductive Health and Research directly from the UN Population Division.

[e] *World malaria report 2005.* Geneva, World Health Organization, United Nations Children's Fund, 2005. Values for Cameroon and Chad have been updated for this report.

[f] *Towards universal access: scaling up priority HIV/AIDS interventions in the health sector.* Geneva, World Health Organization, UNAIDS, United Nations Children's Fund, 2007. See Annex 1: Estimated number of people receiving antiretroviral therapy, people needing antiretroviral therapy and percentage coverage in WHO Member States. Ranges of estimates are available from this document.

[g] PMTCT, preventing mother-to-child transmission. The coverage estimate is calculated by dividing the number of pregnant HIV-infected women who received antiretrovirals for PMTCT by the estimated unrounded number of pregnant HIV-infected women. Source: *Towards universal access: scaling up priority HIV/AIDS interventions in the health sector.* Geneva, World Health Organization, UNAIDS, United Nations Children's Fund, 2007. See Annex 3: Preventing mother-to-child transmission of HIV in low- and middle-income countries, 2005. Ranges of estimates are available from this document.

Children aged <5 years sleeping under insecticide-treated bednets[e]		Antiretroviral therapy coverage		TB detection rate under DOTS[h]	TB treatment success under DOTS[i]	Children aged < 5 years with ARI symptoms taken to facility[j]		Children aged < 5 years with diarrhoea receiving ORT[j]		Children aged < 5 years with fever who received treatment with any antimalarial[e]		Children 6–59 months who received vitamin A supplementation[j]		Births by Caesarean section[h]	
		People with advanced HIV infections[l]	HIV-infected pregnant women for PMTCT[p]												
(%)	Year	(%) Dec 2006	(%) Dec 2005	(%) 2005	(%) 2004 cohort	(%)	Year	(%)	Year	(%)	Year	(%)	Year	(%)	Year
...		...	90	...	...	...		...		...		...		9	1999
...		...	...	19	70	...		...		...		...		...	
...		...	...	...	...	...		...		...		...		17	1997
2	1999	18	6	45	81	56.6	2005	70.0	2005	53.4	1999	41.2	2005	3	1999
...		...	...	85	61	...		...		...		...		23	2000
...		51	...	83	...	...		...		...		...		...	
...		...	...	39	78	...		...		...		...		...	
...		...	...	61	90	...		...		...		...		...	
...		71	...	73	81	...		...		...		...		...	
16	2000	17	7	84	93	71.3	2002	74.0	2002	6.5	2000	...		10	2002
...		0	...	41	82	32.2	1997	64.6	1997	...		...		1	1997
7	2001–2002	35	15	52	83	69.1	2002	66.9	2002	51.9	2001–2002	67.4	2002	2	2001–2002
...		15	9	41	54	49.8	1999	79.7	1999	...		...		7	1999
...		...	...	...	...	...		...		...		...		...	
...		29	11	50	74	...		...		...		...		...	
...		...	...	65	80	...		...		...		...		...	
...		18	6	64	87	...		...		...		...		...	
...		...	...	35	74	...		...		...		...		...	
...		...	...	44	83	...		...		...		...		...	
...		30	4	76	91	...		...		...		...		...	
...		...	...	60	84	...		...		...		...		...	

[h] TB, tuberculosis; DOTS, internationally recommended TB control strategy. The detection rate is the number of new smear-positive cases notified to WHO divided by the estimated number of new smear-positive cases. Source: *Global tuberculosis control: surveillance, planning, financing. WHO report 2007*. Geneva, World Health Organization, 2007 (WHO/HTM/TB/2007.376) (http://www.who.int/tb/publications/global_report).

[i] The treatment success rate is the percentage of new smear-positive patients registered for treatment under DOTS during 2004 who were cured (with laboratory confirmation) or completed their course of treatment. Source: *Global tuberculosis control: surveillance, planning, financing. WHO report 2007*. Geneva, World Health Organization, 2007 (WHO/HTM/TB/2007.376) (http://www.who.int/tb/publications/global_report).

[j] ARI, acute respiratory infection; ORT, oral rehydration therapy. Data compiled by the Department of Child and Adolescent Health and Development, WHO, from *Demographic and Health Surveys: final reports, 2007* (http://www.measuredhs.com/pubs/search/search_results.cfm?Type=5&srchTp=type&newSrch=1, accessed 15 February 2007).

[k] In this case, data do not relate to "skilled health personnel" as defined in the document *Making pregnancy safer: the critical role of the skilled attendant. A joint statement by WHO, ICM and FIGO*. Geneva, World Health Organization, 2004. Further information can be found at http://www.who.int/reproductive-health/global_monitoring/RHRxmls/RHRmainpage.htm.

[l] Excludes Transnistria region.

[m] Covers Northern Sudan and selected sites in Southern Sudan.

[n] See footnote o to the table on Health status: mortality.

Risk factors

Figures have been computed by WHO to ensure comparability; thus they are not necessarily the official statistics of Member States, which may use alternative rigorous methods.

	Member State	WHO region	Children aged <5 years stunted for age[a]		Children aged <5 years underweight for age[a]		Children aged <5 years overweight for age[a]		Low-birthweight newborns[b]	Adults aged ≥15 years who are obese[c]		
			(%)	Year	(%)	Year	(%)	Year	(%)	(%)		Year
			Both sexes		Both sexes		Both sexes		Both sexes 2000–2002	Male	Female	
1	Afghanistan	EMR	53.6	1997	46.2	1997	...	...	...	...	...	
2	Albania	EUR	39.2	2000	17.0	2000	30.0	2000	3	...	...	
3	Algeria	AFR	21.6	2002	10.2	2002	15.4	2002	7	...	...	
4	Andorra	EUR	...		...		...		...	...	...	
5	Angola	AFR	50.8	2001	27.5	2001	5.3	2001	12	...	...	
6	Antigua and Barbuda	AMR	...		...		...		8	...	...	
7	Argentina	AMR	8.2	2004–2005	2.3	2004–2005	9.9	2004–2005	7	...	...	
8	Armenia	EUR	18.2	2005	4.2	2005	11.7	2005	7	...	14.1	2000–2001[m]
9	Australia	WPR	...		...		...		7	19.4	22.0	1999–2000[n]
10	Austria	EUR	...		...		...		7	...	...	
11	Azerbaijan	EUR	24.1	2000	14.0	2000	6.2	2000	11	...	12.4	2001[k]
12	Bahamas	AMR	...		...		...		7	...	...	
13	Bahrain	EMR	...		...		...		8	23.3	34.1	1998–1999[n]
14	Bangladesh	SEAR	50.5	2004	42.7	2004	0.9	2004	30	...	...	
15	Barbados	AMR	...		...		...		10	...	...	
16	Belarus	EUR	...		...		...		5	...	...	
17	Belgium	EUR	...		...		...		8	11.9	13.4	2004[o]
18	Belize	AMR	...		...		...		6	...	...	
19	Benin	AFR	39.1	2001	21.5	2001	3.0	2001	16	...	6.1	2001[m]
20	Bhutan	SEAR	47.7	1999	14.1	1999	3.9	1999	15	...	...	
21	Bolivia	AMR	32.5	2003–2004	5.9	2003–2004	9.2	2003–2004	9	...	15.1	2003[m]
22	Bosnia and Herzegovina	EUR	12.1	2000	4.2	2000	16.3	2000	4	16.5	25.2	2002[n]
23	Botswana	AFR	29.1	2000	10.7	2000	10.4	2000	10	...	...	
24	Brazil	AMR	...		3.7	2002–2003	...		10	8.9	13.1	2002–2003[n]
25	Brunei Darussalam	WPR	...		...		...		10	...	...	
26	Bulgaria	EUR	8.8	2004	1.6	2004	13.6	2004	10	...	...	
27	Burkina Faso	AFR	43.1	2003	35.2	2003	5.4	2003	19	...	2.4	2003[m]
28	Burundi	AFR	63.1	2000	38.9	2000	1.4	2000	16	...	...	
29	Cambodia	WPR	49.2	2000	39.5	2000	4.0	2000	11	...	0.7	2000[m]
30	Cameroon	AFR	35.4	2004	15.1	2004	8.7	2004	11	...	8.2	2004[m]
31	Canada	AMR	...		...		...		6	15.9	13.9	2003[n,o]
32	Cape Verde	AFR	...		...		...		13	...	...	
33	Central African Republic	AFR	44.6	2000	21.8	2000	10.8	2000	14	...	...	
34	Chad	AFR	44.8	2004	33.9	2004	4.4	2004	17	...	...	
35	Chile	AMR	2.7	2006	0.8	2006	11.7	2006	5	19.0	25.0	2003[n]
36	China	WPR	18.6	2002	6.1	2002	6.1	2002	6	2.4	3.4	2002[n]
37	Colombia	AMR	16.2	2005	5.1	2004–2005	4.2	2004–2005	9	8.8	16.6	2005[n]
38	Comoros	AFR	46.9	2000	25.0	2000	21.5	2000	25	...	...	
39	Congo	AFR	31.2	2005	11.8	2005	8.5	2005	...	...	...	
40	Cook Islands	WPR	...		...		...		3	55.7	60.5	2003[n]
41	Costa Rica	AMR	...		...		...		7	...	...	
42	Côte d'Ivoire	AFR	31.5	1998–1999	18.2	1998–1999	4.6	1998–1999	17	...	5.0	1998–1999[m]
43	Croatia	EUR	...		...		...		6	21.6	22.7	2003[n]
44	Cuba	AMR	9.6	2000	4.3	2000	...		6	...	...	
45	Cyprus	EUR	...		...		...		...	...	...	

Access to improved drinking water sources[d]		Access to improved sanitation[d]		Population using solid fuels[a]		Prevalence of current tobacco use (%)[f]					Per capita recorded alcohol consumption[j] (litres of pure alcohol) among adults (≥15 years)	Prevalence of condom use by young people (15–24 years) at higher risk sex[i] (%)		
(%)		(%)		(%)		Adolescents (13–15 years)[jii]		Adults (≥15 years)[h]						
Urban 2004	Rural 2004	Urban 2004	Rural 2004	Urban 2003	Rural 2003	Both sexes	Year	Male	Female	Year	2003	Male	Female	Year
63	31	49	29	...	...	...		...	...		0.01	...	...	
99	94	99	84	...	...	13.0	2004	46.3	3.0	2002[k,l]	2.01	...	...	
88	80	99	82	...	...	...		...	...		0.16	...	...	
100	100	100	100	...	...	...		...	...		...	...	...	
75	40	56	16	...	...	...		...	...		3.86	...	...	
95	89	98	94	...	...	14.1	2004	...	...		5.73	...	...	
98	80	92	83	...	...	...		...	...		8.40	...	...	
99	80	96	61	9	54	7.3	2004	67.5	3.1	2001[m]	1.48	44	...	2000
100	100	100	100	...	...	...		...	...		9.02	...	...	
100	100	100	100	...	...	...		...	...		11.08	...	...	
95	59	73	36	...	...	...		...	...		4.54	...	...	
98	86	100	100	...	...	11.9	2004	...	...		10.40	...	...	
100	...	100	...	...	...	19.9	2002	15.0	3.1	2001	6.98	...	...	
82	72	51	35	54	99	...		58.2	8.2	2003[n]	0.00	...	...	
100	100	99	100	...	...	14.8	2002	...	...		...	...	...	
100	100	93	61	...	...	26.9	2004	...	...		5.53	...	...	
100	100	100	100	...	...	...		28.0	20.0	2001	10.63	...	...	
100	82	71	25	...	...	18.1	2002	...	...		6.25	...	...	
78	57	59	11	88	99	14.5	2003	...	...		1.29	34	19	2001
86	60	65	70	...	...	18.1	2004	...	...		0.23	...	...	
95	68	60	22	5	80	...		...	...		3.23	37	20	2003
99	96	99	92	21	75	...		54.2	34.2	2003[n]	9.05	...	...	
100	90	57	25	...	...	11.3	2001	...	...		4.29	88	75	2000
96	57	83	37	5	53	...		26.3	17.5	2003[n]	5.76	...	...	
...	...	...	...	...	...	...		...	...		0.12	...	...	
100	97	100	96	...	...	34.3	2002	...	...		5.86	...	...	
94	54	42	6	91	100	...		24.2	11.1	2003[n]	5.01	67	54	2003
92	77	47	35	98	100	...		...	...		9.10	...	...	
64	35	53	8	82	99	5.1	2003	...	...		1.48	...	...	
86	44	58	43	62	98	...		...	...		3.77	57	46	2004
100	99	100	99	...	...	...		22.0	18.0	2003[l]	7.80	...	...	
86	73	61	19	...	...	...		...	...		4.78	...	...	
93	61	47	12	...	...	...		...	...		1.53	...	...	
41	43	24	4	95	98	...		18.3	3.7	2003[n]	0.31	25	17	2004
100	58	95	62	...	...	...		48.3	36.8	2003[n]	6.60	...	...	
93	67	69	28	...	...	...		57.4	3.5	2003[n,p]	5.20	...	...	
99	71	96	54	3	48	...		...	...		5.68	...	30	2000
92	82	41	29	46	90	...		27.5	17.0	2003[n,p]	0.31	...	...	
84	27	28	25	84	98	...		16.5	1.7	2003[n,p]	2.60	...	...	
98	88	100	100	...	...	45.1	2003	...	...		3.73	...	...	
100	92	89	97	...	...	18.7	2002	...	...		5.65	...	...	
97	74	46	29	63	95	...		20.7	3.2	2003[n,p]	1.77	...	...	
100	100	100	100	7	24	18.9	2003	31.6	22.9	2003[n]	12.25	...	...	
95	78	99	95	...	...	...		...	...		2.26	...	...	
100	100	100	100	...	...	...		...	...		11.52	...	...	

Risk factors

Figures have been computed by WHO to ensure comparability; thus they are not necessarily the official statistics of Member States, which may use alternative rigorous methods.

	Member State	WHO region	Children aged <5 years stunted for age[a]		Children aged <5 years underweight for age[a]		Children aged <5 years overweight for age[a]		Low-birthweight newborns[b]	Adults aged ≥15 years who are obese[c]		
			(%)	Year	(%)	Year	(%)	Year	(%)	(%)		Year
			Both sexes		Both sexes		Both sexes		Both sexes 2000–2002	Male	Female	
46	Czech Republic	EUR	2.6	2001–2002	2.1	2001–2002	4.4	2001–2002	7	13.7	16.3	2002[n,o]
47	Democratic People's Republic of Korea	SEAR	44.7	2002	17.8	2002	0.9	2002	7	...	...	
48	Democratic Republic of the Congo	AFR	44.4	2001	33.6	2001	6.5	2001	12	...	...	
49	Denmark	EUR	...		...		...		5	9.8	9.1	2000[n,o]
50	Djibouti	EMR	28.6	2002	23.9	2002	...		...	...	...	
51	Dominica	AMR	...		...		...		10	...	...	
52	Dominican Republic	AMR	11.7	2002	4.2	2002	8.6	2002	11	12.7	18.3	1996–1998[n]
53	Ecuador	AMR	29.0	2004	6.2	2004	5.1	2004	16	...	...	
54	Egypt	EMR	23.8	2005	5.4	2005	14.1	2005	12	12.6	33.0	1998–1999[n]
55	El Salvador	AMR	24.6	2002–2003	6.1	2002–2003	5.8	2002–2003	13	...	...	
56	Equatorial Guinea	AFR	42.6	2000	15.7	2000	14.0	2000	13	...	...	
57	Eritrea	AFR	43.7	2002	34.5	2002	1.6	2002	21	...	1.6	2002[m]
58	Estonia	EUR	...		...		...		4	13.7	14.9	2004[n,o]
59	Ethiopia	AFR	50.7	2005	34.6	2005	5.1	2005	15	...	0.3	2000[m]
60	Fiji	WPR	...		...		...		10	9.8	26.4	2002[n]
61	Finland	EUR	...		...		...		4	21.2	23.5	2000–2001[n]
62	France	EUR	...		...		...		7	...	...	
63	Gabon	AFR	26.3	2000–2001	8.8	2000–2001	5.6	2000–2001	14	...	8.2	2000[m]
64	Gambia	AFR	24.1	2000	15.4	2000	3.0	2000	17	...	...	
65	Georgia	EUR	15.2	1999	3.4	1999	17.7	1999	6	...	...	
66	Germany	EUR	...		...		...		7	13.6	12.3	2002–2003[n,o]
67	Ghana	AFR	35.6	2003	18.8	2003	4.5	2003	11	...	8.1	2003[m]
68	Greece	EUR	...		...		...		8	26.0	18.2	2004[n]
69	Grenada	AMR	...		...		...		9	...	...	
70	Guatemala	AMR	54.3	2002	17.7	2002	5.6	2002	13	...	12.2	1998–1999[m]
71	Guinea	AFR	39.3	2005	22.5	2005	5.1	2005	12	...	2.6	1999[m]
72	Guinea-Bissau	AFR	36.1	2000	21.9	2000	5.1	2000	22	...	...	
73	Guyana	AMR	13.8	2000	11.9	2000	5.5	2000	12	...	...	
74	Haiti	AMR	28.3	2000	13.9	2000	3.1	2000	21	...	7.8	2000[m]
75	Honduras	AMR	29.9	2005–2006	8.6	2005–2006	5.8	2005–2006	14	...	...	
76	Hungary	EUR	...		...		...		9	17.1	18.2	2003–2004[n,o]
77	Iceland	EUR	...		...		...		4	12.4	12.3	2002[o]
78	India	SEAR	51.0	1998–1999	44.4	1998–1999	3.6	1998–1999	30	0.3	0.6	1998[n]
79	Indonesia	SEAR	28.6	2004	19.7	2004	5.1	2004	9	1.1	3.6	2001
80	Iran (Islamic Republic of)	EMR	19.7	1998	9.1	1998	7.0	1998	7	5.6	14.2	1999
81	Iraq	EMR	28.3	2000	12.9	2000	5.5	2000	15	...	...	
82	Ireland	EUR	...		...		...		6	14.0	12.0	2002[n,o]
83	Israel	EUR	...		...		...		8	19.8	25.4	1999–2001[n]
84	Italy	EUR	...		...		...		6	9.3	8.7	2003[n,o]
85	Jamaica	AMR	4.5	2004	3.1	2004	7.5	2004	9	...	...	
86	Japan	WPR	...		...		...		8	2.9	3.3	2001
87	Jordan	EMR	12.0	2002	3.6	2002	4.7	2002	10	...	26.3	2002[m]
88	Kazakhstan	EUR	13.9	1999	3.8	1999	5.3	1999	8	...	12.7	1999[m]
89	Kenya	AFR	35.8	2003	16.5	2003	5.8	2003	11	...	6.3	2003[m]
90	Kiribati	WPR	...		...		...		5	...	...	

World Health Statistics 2007

Access to improved drinking water sources[d] (%)		Access to improved sanitation[d] (%)		Population using solid fuels[e] (%)		Prevalence of current tobacco use (%)[f]					Per capita recorded alcohol consumption[i] (litres of pure alcohol) among adults (≥15 years)	Prevalence of condom use by young people (15–24 years) at higher risk sex[j] (%)		
						Adolescents (13–15 years)[g]		Adults (≥15 years)[h]						
Urban 2004	Rural 2004	Urban 2004	Rural 2004	Urban 2003	Rural 2003	Both sexes	Year	Male	Female	Year	2003	Male	Female	Year
100	100	99	97	1	5	34.6	2002	38.9	25.1	2003[n]	12.99	...	...	
100	100	58	60	...	...	...		...	...		3.26	...	...	
82	29	42	25	...	...	...		...	...		1.86	...	...	
100	100	100	100	...	...	...		...	...		11.71	...	...	
76	59	88	50	2	50	14.9	2003	...	...		1.79	...	...	
100	90	86	75	...	...	17.2	2004	...	...		7.50	...	...	
97	91	81	73	7	35	14.9	2004	17.2	12.4	2003[n]	6.66	52	29	2002
97	89	94	82	1	8	...		28.7	7.0	2003[n]	2.36	...	...	
99	97	86	58	0	4	12.6	2005	...	...		0.21	...	...	
94	70	77	39	...	...	19.0	2003	...	...		3.72	...	...	
45	42	60	46	...	...	...		...	...		3.38	...	...	
74	57	32	3	31	97	6.6	2006	...	...		0.59	...	...	
100	99	97	96	10	34	29.5	2003	56.5	24.8	2003[n]	9.00	...	...	
81	11	44	7	78	100	...		7.3	0.6	2003[n]	0.86	30	17	2000
43	51	87	55	...	...	12.2	2005	...	...		1.72	...	...	
100	100	100	100	...	...	...		...	...		9.31	...	...	
100	100	...	...	...	...	...		...	...		11.43	...	...	
95	47	37	30	14	81	...		...	...		8.01	48	33	2000
95	77	72	46	...	...	...		...	...		2.59	...	...	
96	67	96	91	11	78	24.6	2003	60.3	6.2	2003[n]	1.47	...	...	
100	100	100	100	...	...	...		33.2	22.1	2003	11.99	...	...	
88	64	27	11	75	96	11.7	2006	9.9	1.3	2003[n]	1.57	52	33	2003
...	...	...	...	...	...	16.2	2005	...	...		9.01	...	...	
97	93	96	97	...	...	16.7	2004	...	...		6.67	...	...	
99	92	90	82	32	86	16.2	2002	24.4	3.5	2003[n]	1.46	...	...	
78	35	31	11	...	...	...		...	...		0.20	42	27	2005
79	49	57	23	...	...	...		...	...		2.19	...	...	
83	83	86	60	...	...	14.9	2004	...	...		3.84	...	...	
52	56	57	14	91	100	...		...	...		8.30	30	19	2000
95	81	87	54	...	...	...		...	...		2.92	...	...	
100	98	100	85	...	...	27.8	2003	42.7	31.3	2003[n]	13.60	...	...	
100	100	100	100	...	...	...		22.0	23.0	2005	6.99	...	...	
95	83	59	22	22	89	17.5	2004	42.0	8.5	2003[n,p]	0.29	59	51	2001
87	69	73	40	20	83	...		69.0	3.0	2001	0.09	...	...	
99	84	...	...	...	...	13.0	2003	...	...		0.00	...	...	
97	50	95	48	...	...	...		...	...		0.21	...	...	
100	...	...	...	...	...	...		23.7	24.3	2005	13.69	...	...	
100	100	100	...	...	...	...		38.6	22.1	2001[n,q]	2.47	...	...	
100	...	...	...	...	...	...		...	...		8.02	...	...	
98	88	91	69	...	...	19.3	2000	...	...		1.74	...	...	
100	100	100	100	...	...	...		47.9	12.2	2003[l,n]	7.59	...	...	
99	91	94	87	...	...	28.5	2003	50.5	8.3	2002[l,n]	0.31	...	...	
97	73	87	52	1	11	11.4	2004	52.3	9.7	2003[n]	2.96	...	...	
83	46	46	41	17	94	12.7	2001	27.2	1.9	2003[n]	1.51	47	25	2003
77	53	59	22	...	...	...		...	...		0.45	...	...	

Risk factors

Figures have been computed by WHO to ensure comparability; thus they are not necessarily the official statistics of Member States, which may use alternative rigorous methods.

	Member State	WHO region	Children aged <5 years stunted for age[a]		Children aged <5 years underweight for age[a]		Children aged <5 years overweight for age[a]		Low-birthweight newborns[b]	Adults aged ≥15 years who are obese[c]		
			(%)	Year	(%)	Year	(%)	Year	(%)	(%)		Year
			Both sexes		Both sexes		Both sexes		Both sexes 2000–2002	Male	Female	
91	Kuwait	EMR	6.7	1996–1997	1.9	1996–1997	9.2	1996–1997	7	27.6	29.9	1998–2000[r]
92	Kyrgyzstan	EUR	32.6	1997	8.2	1997	9.2	1997	7	...	8.6	1997[m]
93	Lao People's Democratic Republic	WPR	48.2	2000	36.4	2000	2.7	2000	14	0.7	1.6	2000
94	Latvia	EUR	...		...		...		5	11.9	19.5	2004[o]
95	Lebanon	EMR	5.8	1997	4.3	2004	...		6	14.3	18.8	1997[n]
96	Lesotho	AFR	53.0	2000	15.0	2000	21.0	2000	14	...	16.1	2004
97	Liberia	AFR	45.3	1999–2000	22.8	1999–2000	4.6	1999–2000	...	...	...	
98	Libyan Arab Jamahiriya	EMR	...		...		...		7	...	...	
99	Lithuania	EUR	...		...		...		4	14.2	16.9	2004[n,o]
100	Luxembourg	EUR	...		...		...		8	...	...	
101	Madagascar	AFR	52.8	2003–2004	36.8	2003–2004	6.2	2003–2004	14	...	1.0	2003–2004
102	Malawi	AFR	52.5	2004–2005	18.4	2004–2005	10.2	2004–2005	16	...	2.1	2000[m]
103	Malaysia	WPR	20.0	1999	16.2	1999	5.9	1999	10	...	...	
104	Maldives	SEAR	31.9	2001	25.7	2001	3.9	2001	22	...	...	
105	Mali	AFR	42.7	2001	30.1	2001	3.1	2001	23	...	3.7	2001[m]
106	Malta	EUR	...		...		...		6	25.0	21.3	2002[n,o]
107	Marshall Islands	WPR	...		...		...		12	...	...	
108	Mauritania	AFR	39.5	2000–2001	30.4	2000–2001	3.8	2000–2001	...	...	16.7	2000–2001[m]
109	Mauritius	AFR	...		...		...		13	7.5	19.8	1998[n]
110	Mexico	AMR	15.5	2006	3.4	2006	7.6	2006	9	18.6	28.1	2000[n]
111	Micronesia (Federated States of)	WPR	...		...		...		18	...	...	
112	Monaco	EUR	...		...		...		...	...	...	
113	Mongolia	WPR	23.5	2004	4.8	2004	6.1	2004	8	7.2	12.5	2006
114	Montenegro	EUR	13.0	2000	2.3	2000	...		0	...	...	
115	Morocco	EMR	23.1	2003–2004	9.9	2003–2004	13.3	2003–2004	11	8.2	21.7	2000[n]
116	Mozambique	AFR	47.0	2003	21.2	2003	6.3	2003	14	...	3.9	2003
117	Myanmar	SEAR	40.6	2003	29.6	2003	2.4	2003	15	...	...	
118	Namibia	AFR	29.5	2000	20.3	2000	3.3	2000	14	...	...	
119	Nauru	WPR	...		...		...		...	55.7	60.5	2004[n]
120	Nepal	SEAR	57.1	2001	43.0	2001	0.7	2001	21	...	1.0	2001
121	Netherlands	EUR	...		...		...		...	10.2	11.9	1998–2001
122	New Zealand	WPR	...		...		...		6	21.9	23.2	2002–2003
123	Nicaragua	AMR	25.2	2001	7.8	2001	7.1	2001	12	...	18.0	2001[m]
124	Niger	AFR	54.2	2000	43.6	2000	1.6	2000	17	...	1.6	1998
125	Nigeria	AFR	43.0	2003	27.2	2003	6.2	2003	14	...	5.8	2003[m]
126	Niue	WPR	...		...		...		...	...	...	
127	Norway	EUR	...		...		...		5	6.8	5.8	1998[n,o]
128	Oman	EMR	15.9	1998	13.1	1998	1.7	1998	8	...	...	
129	Pakistan	EMR	41.5	2001	31.3	2001	4.8	2001	19	...	...	
130	Palau	WPR	...		...		...		9	...	...	
131	Panama	AMR	21.5	1997	6.3	1997	6.2	1997	10	...	...	
132	Papua New Guinea	WPR	43.9	2005	18.1	2005	...		11	...	...	
133	Paraguay	AMR	...		...		...		9	...	...	
134	Peru	AMR	31.3	2000	5.2	2000	11.8	2000	11	11.5	19.9	2000[n]
135	Philippines	WPR	33.8	2003	20.7	2003	2.4	2003	20	3.0	6.2	1998[n]

Access to improved drinking water sources[d] (%)		Access to improved sanitation[d] (%)		Population using solid fuels[e] (%)		Prevalence of current tobacco use (%)[f]					Per capita recorded alcohol consumption[i] (litres of pure alcohol) among adults (≥15 years)	Prevalence of condom use by young people (15–24 years) at higher risk sex[j] (%)		
						Adolescents (13–15 years)[g]		Adults (≥15 years)[h]						
Urban 2004	Rural 2004	Urban 2004	Rural 2004	Urban 2003	Rural 2003	Both sexes	Year	Male	Female	Year	2003	Male	Female	Year
...	...	...	...	...	...	21.1	2001	...	...		0.03	...	...	
98	66	75	51	...	...	7.2	2004	45.0	1.6	2005	3.63	...	...	
79	43	67	20	88	99	...		66.1	15.4	2003[n]	6.91	...	...	
100	96	82	71	3	26	34.2	2002	64.3	24.1	2003[n]	9.61	...	...	
100	100	100	87	...	...	59.7	2005	...	...		3.24	...	...	
92	76	61	32	...	...	20.3	2002	...	...		1.82	48	50	2004
72	52	49	7	...	...	...		...	...		3.82	...	...	
...	...	97	96	...	...	12.7	2003	...	...		0.01	...	...	
...	...	...	...	...	...	32.1	2005	...	...		9.89	...	...	
100	100	100	100	...	...	...		36.0	26.0	2004	15.56	...	...	
77	35	48	26	...	...	...		...	...		1.59	12	5	2003
98	68	62	61	90	99	...		25.3	5.8	2003[n]	1.41	47	35	2004
100	96	95	93	1	2	16.7	2004	53.2	2.6	2003[n]	1.06	...	...	
98	76	100	42	...	...	...		27.3	2.2	2001[l,n]	...	...	...	
78	36	59	39	99	100	...		24.7	3.0	2003[n]	0.50	30	14	2001
100	100	100	...	...	...	...		...	...		6.02	...	...	
82	96	93	58	...	...	...		...	...		...	...	...	
59	44	49	8	35	84	24.7	2001	29.6	4.7	2003[n]	0.01	...	...	
100	100	95	94	0	2	13.2	2003	42.7	2.8	2003[n]	3.03	...	...	
100	87	91	41	4	45	...		35.9	15.0	2003[n]	4.57	...	...	
95	94	61	14	...	...	...		...	...		1.23	...	...	
100	...	100	...	...	...	...		...	...		...	...	...	
87	30	75	37	...	...	14.9	2003	...	...		2.83	...	...	
...	...	...	...	...	...	...		...	...		...	...	...	
99	56	88	52	0	13	10.8	2001	32.1	0.2	2003[n]	0.45	...	...	
72	26	53	19	...	...	...		...	...		0.52	33	29	2003
80	77	88	72	88	100	13.4	2004	48.7	13.7	2003[n]	0.33	...	...	
98	81	50	13	24	84	25.8	2004	28.3	12.4	2003[n]	5.97	69	48	2000
...	...	...	...	...	...	...		...	...		0.87	...	...	
96	89	62	30	27	90	...		42.0	21.1	2003[n]	0.19	...	...	
100	100	100	100	...	...	...		...	...		9.68	...	...	
100	...	...	...	...	...	...		25.1	24.8	2001[l]	9.68	...	...	
90	63	56	34	40	93	22.3	2003	...	...		2.48	...	17	2001
80	36	43	4	95	98	18.4	2001	...	...		0.05	...	...	
67	31	53	36	...	...	...		...	0.0	2003[l,m]	10.57	46	24	2003
100	100	100	100	...	...	...		...	...		9.47	...	...	
100	100	100	100	...	...	...		...	...		5.50	...	...	
...	...	97	...	...	...	14.3	2002	...	...		0.26	...	...	
96	89	92	41	66	92	...		33.7	6.2	2003[n]	0.01	...	...	
79	94	96	52	...	...	33.1	2005	...	...		...	...	...	
99	79	89	51	...	...	18.6	2002	...	...		5.98	...	...	
88	32	67	41	34	98	...		...	...		1.62	...	...	
99	68	94	61	30	83	...		41.4	13.2	2003[n]	3.73	...	...	
89	65	74	32	13	90	21.2	2003	...	...		3.83	...	25	2004
87	82	80	59	27	70	15.9	2004	57.6	12.3	2003[n]	3.51	...	...	

Risk factors

Figures have been computed by WHO to ensure comparability; thus they are not necessarily the official statistics of Member States, which may use alternative rigorous methods.

	Member State	WHO region	Children aged <5 years stunted for age[a]		Children aged <5 years underweight for age[a]		Children aged <5 years overweight for age[a]		Low-birthweight newborns[b]	Adults aged ≥15 years who are obese[c]		
			(%)	Year	(%)	Year	(%)	Year	(%)	(%)		Year
			Both sexes		Both sexes		Both sexes		Both sexes 2000–2002	Male	Female	
136	Poland	EUR	...		...		...		6	15.7	19.9	2000[n]
137	Portugal	EUR	...		...		...		8	...	...	
138	Qatar	EMR	...		...		...		10	...	...	
139	Republic of Korea	WPR	...		...		...		4	1.7	3.0	1998[n]
140	Republic of Moldova	EUR	11.3	2005	3.2	2005	9.1	2005	5	...	...	
141	Romania	EUR	12.8	2002	3.5	2002	8.3	2002	9	9.1	19.1	1997
142	Russian Federation	EUR	...		...		...		6	...	...	
143	Rwanda	AFR	48.3	2000	20.3	2000	7.2	2000	9	...	...	
144	Saint Kitts and Nevis	AMR	...		...		...		9	...	...	
145	Saint Lucia	AMR	...		...		...		8	...	...	
146	Saint Vincent and the Grenadines	AMR	...		...		...		10	...	...	
147	Samoa	WPR	8.7	1999	2.1	1999	6.8	1999	4	44.9	66.3	2002[n]
148	San Marino	EUR	...		...		...		...	...	...	
149	Sao Tome and Principe	AFR	35.2	2000	10.1	2000	9.2	2000	...	...	...	
150	Saudi Arabia	EMR	...		...		...		11	26.4	44.0	1995–2000[n]
151	Senegal	AFR	20.1	2005	14.5	2005	2.4	2005	18	...	...	
152	Serbia	EUR	9.8	2000	2.1	2000	...		0	...	...	
153	Seychelles	AFR	...		...		...		...	15.0	35.2	2004[n]
154	Sierra Leone	AFR	38.4	2000	24.7	2000	4.7	2000	...	...	...	
155	Singapore	WPR	4.4	2000	3.3	2000	2.6	2000	8	5.3	6.7	1998[n]
156	Slovakia	EUR	...		...		...		7	...	...	
157	Slovenia	EUR	...		...		...		6	16.5	13.8	2001[n,o]
158	Solomon Islands	WPR	...		...		...		13	...	...	
159	Somalia	EMR	29.0	2000	23.0	2000	...		...	...	...	
160	South Africa	AFR	30.9	1999	9.6	1999	9.3	1999	15	9.3	30.1	1998
161	Spain	EUR	...		...		...		6	13.0	13.5	2003
162	Sri Lanka	SEAR	18.4	2000	22.8	2000	1.0	2000	22	...	...	
163	Sudan	EMR	47.6	2000	38.4	2000	5.2	2000	31	...	...	
164	Suriname	AMR	14.5	1999–2000	11.4	1999–2000	2.9	1999–2000	13	...	...	
165	Swaziland	AFR	36.6	2000	9.1	2000	14.9	2000	9	...	...	
166	Sweden	EUR	...		...		...		4	10.4	9.5	2002–2003[n,o]
167	Switzerland	EUR	...		...		...		6	7.9	7.5	2002[o]
168	Syrian Arab Republic	EMR	24.1	2000	9.1	2001	...		6	...	...	
169	Tajikistan	EUR	42.0	2003	...		...		15	...	...	
170	Thailand	SEAR	15.5	2006	7.3	2006	10.4	2006	9	...	...	
171	The former Yugoslav Republic of Macedonia	EUR	1.2	2004	1.2	2004	7.9	2004	5	...	10.7	1999[k,n]
172	Timor-Leste	SEAR	55.7	2002	40.6	2002	5.7	2002	10	...	...	
173	Togo	AFR	29.8	1998	23.2	1998	2.6	1998	15	...	...	
174	Tonga	WPR	...		...		...		...	...	...	
175	Trinidad and Tobago	AMR	5.3	2000	4.4	2000	4.9	2000	23	...	...	
176	Tunisia	EMR	16.0	2000	4.4	2000	7.3	1996–1997	7	6.4	22.7	1996–1997[n]
177	Turkey	EUR	19.1	1998	7.0	1998	4.0	1998	16	12.9	29.9	1997[n]
178	Turkmenistan	EUR	27.7	2000	10.0	2000	...		6	...	10.3	2000[m]
179	Tuvalu	WPR	...		...		...		5	...	...	
180	Uganda	AFR	44.8	2000–2001	19.0	2000–2001	4.9	2000–2001	12	...	...	

WORLD HEALTH STATISTICS 2007

Access to improved drinking water sources[d] (%)		Access to improved sanitation[d] (%)		Population using solid fuels[e] (%)		Prevalence of current tobacco use (%)[f]					Per capita recorded alcohol consumption[i] (litres of pure alcohol) among adults (≥15 years)	Prevalence of condom use by young people (15–24 years) at higher risk sex[j] (%)		
						Adolescents (13–15 years)[g]		Adults (≥15 years)[h]						
Urban 2004	Rural 2004	Urban 2004	Rural 2004	Urban 2003	Rural 2003	Both sexes	Year	Male	Female	Year	2003	Male	Female	Year
100	...	...	...	...	...	19.5	2003	...	...		8.09	...	...	
...	...	...	...	...	...	...		...	...		11.54	...	...	
100	100	100	100	...	...	16.6	2004	...	...		4.40	...	...	
97	71	...	...	...	...	10.2	2005	...	...		7.87	...	...	
97	88	86	52	...	...	16.0	2004	...	...		13.18	63	44	2005
91	16	89	...	3	42	18.3	2004	33.2	10.3	2003	9.74	...	...	
100	88	93	70	7	21	27.3	2004	56.7	11.4	2003[n,p]	10.32	...	...	
92	69	56	38	98	100	...		...	...		6.93	41	28	2004
99	99	96	96	...	...	16.6	2002	...	...		6.73	...	...	
98	98	89	89	...	...	13.4	2000	...	...		11.48	...	...	
...	93	...	96	...	...	21.9	2000	...	...		7.00	...	...	
90	87	100	100	...	...	...		...	...		...	...	...	
...	...	...	...	...	...	...		...	...		...	...	...	
89	73	32	20	...	...	...		...	...		6.95	...	...	
97	...	100	...	...	...	...		...	...		0.00	...	...	
92	60	79	34	24	80	16.6	2002	24.1	1.9	2003[n]	0.46	54	34	2005
...	...	...	...	...	...	...		...	...		...	...	...	
100	75	...	100	...	...	28.9	2002	...	...		3.36	...	...	
75	46	53	30	...	...	...		...	...		6.39	...	...	
100	...	100	...	...	...	9.1	2000	...	...		2.17	...	...	
100	99	100	98	2	7	27.3	2003	41.0	23.1	2003[n]	10.35	...	...	
...	...	...	...	...	...	23.6	2003	28.5	19.1	2003[n]	6.74	...	...	
94	65	98	18	...	...	...		...	...		0.97	...	...	
32	27	48	14	...	...	...		...	...		0.00	...	...	
99	73	79	46	7	40	23.6	2002	37.0	11.2	2003[n]	6.72	...	...	
100	100	100	100	1	5	...		40.5	27.1	2003[n]	11.68	...	...	
98	74	98	89	27	77	8.0	2003	39.7	2.9	2003[n]	0.28	...	...	
78	64	50	24	...	...	14.0	2005	...	...		0.30	...	...	
98	73	99	76	...	...	10.5	2004	...	...		...	...	...	
87	54	59	44	23	82	11.5	2001	15.1	3.2	2003[n]	4.60	...	...	
100	100	100	100	...	...	...		...	...		5.96	...	...	
100	100	100	100	...	...	...		...	...		10.83	...	...	
98	87	99	81	...	...	20.0	2002	...	...		0.49	...	...	
92	48	70	45	33	90	5.1	2004	...	...		0.39	...	...	
98	100	98	99	...	...	15.7	2005	48.5	2.9	2001[l]	5.59	...	...	
...	...	...	...	...	...	9.0	2003	...	...		5.69	...	...	
77	56	66	33	...	...	...		...	...		...	...	...	
80	36	71	15	...	...	16.1	2002	...	...		1.24	...	...	
100	100	98	96	...	...	...		...	...		0.75	...	...	
92	88	100	100	...	...	14.3	2000	...	...		4.17	...	...	
99	82	96	65	3	8	15.2	2001	53.0	2.2	2003[n]	1.23	...	...	
98	93	96	72	...	...	8.4	2003	50.7	18.6	2003[n]	1.37	...	...	
93	54	77	50	0	1	...		...	...		1.18	...	...	
94	92	93	84	...	...	...		...	...		1.37	...	...	
87	56	54	41	85	99	...		25.2	3.3	2001[m]	17.64	55	53	2004

Risk factors

Figures have been computed by WHO to ensure comparability; thus they are not necessarily the official statistics of Member States, which may use alternative rigorous methods.

	Member State	WHO region	Children aged <5 years stunted for age[a]		Children aged <5 years underweight for age[a]		Children aged <5 years overweight for age[a]		Low-birthweight newborns[b]	Adults aged ≥15 years who are obese[c]		
			(%)	Year	(%)	Year	(%)	Year	(%)	(%)		Year
			Both sexes		Both sexes		Both sexes		Both sexes 2000–2002	Male	Female	
181	Ukraine	EUR	5.6	2002	4.1	2000	26.5	2000	5	...	...	
182	United Arab Emirates	EMR	...		...		...		15	25.6	39.9	1999–2000[n]
183	United Kingdom	EUR	...		...		...		8	...	...	
184	United Republic of Tanzania	AFR	44.4	2004–2005	16.7	2004–2005	4.9	2004–2005	13	...	4.4	2004–2005
185	United States of America	AMR	3.3	1999–2002	1.1	1999–2002	7.0	1999–2002	8	31.1	33.2	2003–2004[n]
186	Uruguay	AMR	13.9	2004	6.0	2004	9.4	2004	8	17.0	18.0	1998[n]
187	Uzbekistan	EUR	26.2	2002	6.2	2002	...		7	5.4	7.1	2002[m]
188	Vanuatu	WPR	...		...		...		6	12.2	19.6	1998[n]
189	Venezuela (Bolivarian Republic of)	AMR	16.7	2000	4.8	2000	5.7	2000	7	...	...	
190	Viet Nam	WPR	43.4	2000	26.7	2000	2.5	2000	9	...	...	
191	Yemen	EMR	59.8	2003	42.7	2003	3.7	1997	32	...	...	
192	Zambia	AFR	52.5	2001–2002	23.3	2001–2002	5.9	2001–2002	12	...	3.0	2001–2002[m]
193	Zimbabwe	AFR	33.7	1999	11.5	1999	10.6	1999	11	...	7.5	1999[m]
194	The former state union of Serbia and Montenegro[s]	EUR	...		...		...		4	14.4	20.0	2000[n]
	Region											
	African Region	AFR	43.2	2005	23.1	2005	...		14	...	...	
	Region of the Americas	AMR	14.2	2005	4.9	2005	...		9	...	...	
	South-East Asia Region	SEAR	41.6	2005	33.3	2005	...		26	...	...	
	European Region	EUR	...	2005	...	2005	...		8	...	...	
	Eastern Mediterranean Region	EMR	24.9	2005	15.1	2005	...		17	...	...	
	Western Pacific Region	WPR	14.5	2005	6.2	2005	...		8	...	...	
	Global		30.0	2005	17.8	2005	...		16	...	...	

... Data not available or not applicable; AFR, African Region; AMR, Region of the Americas; SEAR, South-East Asia Region; EUR, European Region; EMR, Eastern Mediterranean Region; WPR, Western Pacific Region.

The global values for rates and ratios are weighted averages; for absolute numbers they are the sums of all WHO regions.

[a] *Global database on child growth and malnutrition* [online database]. Geneva, World Health Organization, 2007 (http://www.who.int/nutgrowthdb/database/en).

[b] United Nations Children's Fund, World Health Organization. *Low birthweight: country, regional and global estimates.* New York, UNICEF, 2004 (http://www.who.int/reproductive-health/publications/low_birthweight/low_birthweight_estimates.pdf).

[c] Comparisons between countries may be limited owing to differences in sample characteristics or survey years. Source: *Global database on body mass index (BMI)* [online database]. Geneva, World Health Organization, 2006 (http//www.who.int/bmi).

[d] World Health Organization, United Nations Children's Fund. *Joint monitoring programme for water supply and sanitation* [online database]. Geneva, WHO, UNICEF, 2006 (http://www.wssinfo.org/en/wecome.html).

[e] Estimates were made by WHO's Department of Public Health and Environment based on Rehfuess E, Mehta S, Prüss-Üstün. Assessing household solid fuel use: multiple implications for the Millennium Development Goals. *Environmental Health Perspectives*, 2006, 114:373-378 (http://www.who.int/indoorair/mdg/en).

[f] For adolescents, data relate to daily or occasional tobacco use (smoking, or using oral tobacco or snuff); for adults they relate to daily or occasional tobacco smoking. Comparisons between countries may be limited owing to differences in definitions, sample characteristics or survey years.

[g] *WHO global InfoBase online tool.* Geneva, World Health Organization, 2007 (http://www.who.int/ncd_surveillance/infobase/en).

Access to improved drinking water sources[d] (%)		Access to improved sanitation[d] (%)		Population using solid fuels[e] (%)		Prevalence of current tobacco use (%)[f]					Per capita recorded alcohol consumption[i] (litres of pure alcohol) among adults (≥15 years)	Prevalence of condom use by young people (15–24 years) at higher risk sex[j] (%)		
						Adolescents (13–15 years)[l,c]		Adults (≥15 years)[h]						
Urban 2004	Rural 2004	Urban 2004	Rural 2004	Urban 2003	Rural 2003	Both sexes	Year	Male	Female	Year	2003	Male	Female	Year
99	91	98	93	5	10	26.0	2005	66.8	19.9	2005[o]	6.09	...	...	
100	100	98	95	1	0	18.5	2002	32.4	3.1	2003[n]	0.02	...	...	
100	100	...	...	...	...	...		...	...		11.75	...	...	
85	49	53	43	...	...	...		...	...		5.45	46	34	2004
100	100	100	100	...	...	23.1	2000	24.1	19.2	2003[n]	8.61	...	...	
100	100	100	99	0	7	...		38.5	28.2	2003[n]	7.74	...	...	
95	75	78	61	...	...	...		24.1	0.9	2002[k,m]	1.51	50	...	2002
86	52	78	42	...	...	...		...	...		0.75	...	...	
85	70	71	48	...	...	...		...	...		6.67	...	...	
99	80	92	50	43	78	...		51.1	2.5	2003[n]	0.85	68	...	2005
71	65	86	28	3	53	17.7	2003	...	...		0.04	...	...	
90	40	59	52	68	99	...		23.3	5.7	2003[n]	2.40	42	33	2001
98	72	63	47	26	94	...		26.2	3.1	2003[n]	4.41	...	...	
99	86	97	77	...	...	...		...	...		...	...	...	
82	42	57	30	...	...	...		...	...		4.47	...	...	
98	82	91	66	...	...	...		...	...		6.66	...	...	
92	81	64	31	...	...	...		...	...		0.52	...	...	
99	86	96	77	...	...	...		...	...		8.84	...	...	
94	77	88	43	...	...	...		...	...		0.19	...	...	
94	69	76	34	...	...	...		...	...		5.19	...	...	
95	73	80	39	...	...	...		...	...		4.41	...	...	

[h] Sources: *WHO global InfoBase online tool*. Geneva, World Health Organization, 2007 (also available at http://www.who.int/ncd_surveillance/infobase/en); Ustun TB et al. The World Health Surveys. In: Murray CJL, Evans D, eds. *Health systems performance assessment: debates, methods and empricism*. Geneva, World Health Organization, 2003:797–808; World Health Survey, Geneva, World Health Organization, 2007 (http://www.who.int/healthinfo/survey/en).

[i] *Global alcohol database* [online database]. Geneva, World Health Organization (http://www.who.int/globalatlas/LoginManagement/autologins/gad_login.asp).

[j] *2006 report on the global AIDS epidemic*. Geneva, Joint United Nations Programme on HIV/AIDS, World Health Organization, 2006. See Annex 2: HIV and AIDS estimates and data, 2005 and 2003.

[k] Upper age limit = 45 years.

[l] Cigarettes are the only smoked tobacco product under consideration.

[m] Upper age limit = 50 years.

[n] Lower age limit > 15 years.

[o] Self-reported data.

[p] Sample is not necessarily nationally representative.

[q] Upper age limit = 65 years.

[r] Lower age limit < 15 years.

[s] See footnote o to the table on Health status: mortality.

Health systems

Figures have been computed by WHO to ensure comparability; thus they are not necessarily the official statistics of Member States, which may use alternative rigorous methods.

	Member State	WHO region	Physicians			Nurses			Midwives			Dentists		
			Number	Density per 1000 population	Year	Number	Density per 1000 population	Year	Number	Density per 1000 population	Year	Number	Density per 1000 population	Year
1	Afghanistan	EMR	4 104	0.19	2001	4 752	0.22	2001	...	...		630	0.03	2001
2	Albania	EUR	4 100	1.31	2002	11 473	3.62	2003				1 390	0.45	1998
3	Algeria	AFR	35 368	1.13	2002	62 177	1.99	2002	7 572	0.24	2002	9 553	0.31	2002
4	Andorra	EUR	244	3.70	2003	205	3.11	2003	10	0.15	2003	44	0.67	2003
5	Angola	AFR	1 165	0.08	2004	18 485	1.31	2004	...	...		222	0.02	2004
6	Antigua and Barbuda	AMR	12	0.17	1999	233	3.28	1999	...	...		13	0.19	1997
7	Argentina	AMR	108 800	3.01	1998	29 000	0.80	1998	...	...		28 900	0.80	1998
8	Armenia	EUR	10 983	3.59	2003	13 320	4.35	2003	1 433	0.47	2003	802	0.26	2003
9	Australia	WPR	47 875	2.47	2001	176 188	9.10	2001	11 649	0.60	2001	21 296	1.10	2001
10	Austria	EUR	27 413	3.38	2003	76 161	9.38	2003	1 671	0.21	2003	4 037	0.50	2003
11	Azerbaijan	EUR	29 687	3.55	2003	59 531	7.11	2003	9 803	1.17	2003	2 272	0.27	2003
12	Bahamas	AMR	312	1.05	1998	1 323	4.47	1998	...	...		21	0.07	1998
13	Bahrain	EMR	803	1.09	2004	2 989	4.04	2004	560	0.76	2004	342	0.46	2004
14	Bangladesh	SEAR	38 485	0.26	2004	20 334	0.14	2004	26 460	0.18	2004	2 537	0.02	2004
15	Barbados	AMR	322	1.21	1999	988	3.70	1999	...	...		63	0.24	1999
16	Belarus	EUR	45 027	4.55	2003	115 116	11.63	2003	5 182	0.52	2003	4 315	0.44	2003
17	Belgium	EUR	46 268	4.49	2002	60 142	5.83	2003	6 603	0.64	2001	8 322	0.81	2002
18	Belize	AMR	251	1.05	2000	303	1.26	2000	...	...		32	0.13	2000
19	Benin	AFR	311	0.04	2004	4 965	0.72	2004	824	0.12	2004	12	0.00	2004
20	Bhutan	SEAR	118	0.05	2004	330	0.14	2004	185	0.08	2004	58	0.02	2004
21	Bolivia	AMR	10 329	1.22	2001	18 535	2.19	2001	96	0.01	2001	5 997	0.71	2001
22	Bosnia and Herzegovina	EUR	5 576	1.34	2003	17 170	4.13	2003	1 229	0.30	2003	690	0.17	2003
23	Botswana	AFR	715	0.40	2004	4 753	2.65	2004	...	...		38	0.02	2004
24	Brazil	AMR	198 153	1.15	2000	659 111	3.84	2000	...	...		190 448	1.11	2000
25	Brunei Darussalam	WPR	336	1.01	2000	892	2.67	2000	404	1.21	2000	48	0.14	2000
26	Bulgaria	EUR	28 128	3.56	2003	29 650	3.75	2003	3 456	0.44	2003	6 475	0.82	2003
27	Burkina Faso	AFR	708	0.05	2004	4 268	0.32	2004	2 289	0.17	2004	58	0.00	2004
28	Burundi	AFR	200	0.03	2004	1 337	0.19	2004	11	0.00	2004	14	0.00	2004
29	Cambodia	WPR	2 047	0.16	2000	8 085	0.61	2000	3 040	0.23	2000	209	0.02	2000
30	Cameroon	AFR	3 124	0.19	2004	25 997	1.60	2004	45	0.00	2004	147	0.01	2004
31	Canada	AMR	66 583	2.14	2003	309 576	9.95	2003	...	...		18 265	0.59	2003
32	Cape Verde	AFR	231	0.49	2004	410	0.87	2004	...	...		11	0.02	2004
33	Central African Republic	AFR	331	0.08	2004	908	0.23	2004	705	0.18	2004	13	0.00	2004
34	Chad	AFR	345	0.04	2004	2 146	0.24	2004	353	0.04	2004	15	0.00	2004
35	Chile	AMR	17 250	1.09	2003	10 000	0.63	2003	...	...		6 750	0.43	2003
36	China	WPR	1 364 000	1.06	2001	1 358 000	1.05	2001	42 000	0.03	2001	136 520	0.11	2001
37	Colombia	AMR	58 761	1.35	2002	23 940	0.55	2002	...	...		33 951	0.78	2002
38	Comoros	AFR	115	0.15	2004	481	0.61	2004	107	0.14	2004	29	0.04	2004
39	Congo	AFR	756	0.20	2004	3 214	0.84	2004	458	0.12	2004	12	0.00	2004
40	Cook Islands	WPR	14	0.78	2001	49	2.72	2001	3	0.17	2001	10	0.56	2001
41	Costa Rica	AMR	5 204	1.32	2000	3 631	0.92	2000	22	0.01	2000	1 905	0.48	2000
42	Côte d'Ivoire	AFR	2 081	0.12	2004	7 773	0.46	2004	2 407	0.14	2004	339	0.02	2004
43	Croatia	EUR	10 820	2.44	2003	22 372	5.05	2003	1 476	0.33	2003	3 085	0.70	2003
44	Cuba	AMR	66 567	5.91	2002	83 880	7.44	2002	...	...		9 841	0.87	2002
45	Cyprus	EUR	1 864	2.34	2002	2 994	3.76	2002	...	...		650	0.82	2002
46	Czech Republic	EUR	35 960	3.51	2003	99 351	9.71	2003	4 772	0.47	2003	6 737	0.66	2003
47	Democratic People's Republic of Korea	SEAR	74 597	3.29	2003	87 330	3.85	2003	6 084	0.27	2003	8 315	0.37	2003
48	Democratic Republic of the Congo	AFR	5 827	0.11	2004	28 789	0.53	2004	...	...		159	0.00	2004
49	Denmark	EUR	15 653	2.93	2002	55 425	10.36	2002	1 200	0.22	2002	4 437	0.83	2002
50	Djibouti	EMR	129	0.18	2004	185	0.26	2004	111	0.16	2004	10	0.01	2004
51	Dominica	AMR	38	0.50	1997	317	4.17	1997	...	...		4	0.05	1997
52	Dominican Republic	AMR	15 670	1.88	2000	15 352	1.84	2000	...	...		7 000	0.84	2000
53	Ecuador	AMR	18 335	1.48	2000	19 549	1.57	2000	1 037	0.08	2000	2 062	0.17	2000
54	Egypt	EMR	38 485	0.54	2003	144 984	1.98	2004	1 777	0.02	2004	9 917	0.14	2004
55	El Salvador	AMR	7 938	1.24	2002	5 103	0.80	2002	...	...		3 465	0.54	2002

WORLD HEALTH STATISTICS 2007

Human resources for health[a]																		
Pharmacists			Public and environmental health workers			Community health workers			Laboratory health workers			Other health workers			Health management and support workers			
Number	Density per 1 000 population	Year	Number	Density per 1 000 population	Year	Number	Density per 1 000 population	Year	Number	Density per 1 000 population	Year	Number	Density per 1 000 population	Year	Number	Density per 1 000 population	Year
525	0.02	2001	...	...		...	...		...	...		...	...		...	...	
...	...		...	...		...	...		...	...		...	...		...	...	
6 333	0.20	2002	2 534	0.08	2002	1 062	0.03	2002	8 838	0.28	2002	5 654	0.18	2002	60 316	1.93	2002
68	1.03	2003	...	...		...	...		...	...		...	...		...	...	
919	0.07	2004	...	...		...	...		2 029	0.14	2004	294	0.02	2004	256	0.02	2004
...	...		...	...		...	...		...	...		...	...		...	...	
15 300	0.42	1998	...	...		...	...		...	...		...	...		...	...	
126	0.04	2003	...	...		...	...		...	...		...	...		...	...	
13 956	0.72	2001				3 812	0.20	2001	8 326	0.43	2001	38 339	1.98	2001	488 313	25.23	2001
4 869	0.60	2003	...	...		...	...		...	...		...	...		...	...	
1 842	0.22	2003	...	...		...	...		...	...		...	...		...	...	
...	...		...	...		...	...		...	...		...	...		...	...	
460	0.62	2004	294	0.40	2004		0.00	2004	479	0.65	2004	1 278	1.73	2004	1 697	2.30	2004
9 411	0.06	2004	5 743	0.04	2004	46 202	0.31	2004	3 794	0.03	2004	5 847	0.04	2004	...	...	
...	...		...	...		...	...		...	...		...	...		...	...	
2 901	0.29	2003	...	...		...	...		...	...		...	...		...	...	
11 775	1.14	2002	...	...		...	...		...	...		...	...		...	...	
...	...		...	...		...	...		...	...		...	...		...	...	
11	0.00	2004	178	0.03	2004	88	0.01	2004	477	0.07	2004	130	0.02	2004	3 279	0.47	2004
79	0.03	2004	71	0.03	2004	464	0.20	2004	136	0.06	2004	143	0.06	2004	1 197	0.51	2004
4 670	0.55	2001	...	...		1 579	0.19	2001	...	...		3 399	0.40	2001	8 069	0.95	2001
363	0.09	2003	...	...		...	...		...	...		...	...		...	...	
333	0.19	2004	172	0.10	2004	...	...		277	0.15	2004	829	0.46	2004	...	...	
51 317	0.30	2000	167 080	0.97	2000	...	...		89 677	0.52	2000	191 518	1.11	2000	839 376	4.89	2000
90	0.27	2000	...	...		...	...		...	...		...	...		...	...	
1 020	0.13	2001	...	...		...	...		...	...		...	...		...	...	
343	0.03	2004	46	0.00	2004	1 406	0.10	2004	418	0.03	2004	1 755	0.13	2004	210	0.02	2004
76	0.01	2004	...	...		657	0.09	2004	147	0.02	2004	1 186	0.17	2004	2 087	0.30	2004
564	0.04	2000	...	...		...	...		...	...		...	...		...	...	
700	0.04	2004	28	0.00	2004	...	...		1 793	0.11	2004	16	0.00	2004	5 902	0.36	2004
20 765	0.67	2003	...	...		...	...		...	...		...	...		...	...	
43	0.09	2004	9	0.02	2004	65	0.14	2004	78	0.16	2004	42	0.09	2004	74	0.16	2004
17	0.00	2004	55	0.01	2004	211	0.05	2004	48	0.01	2004	461	0.12	2004	167	0.04	2004
37	0.00	2004	230	0.03	2004	268	0.03	2004	317	0.04	2004	153	0.02	2004	1 502	0.17	2004
...	...		...	...		...	...		...	...		...	...		...	...	
359 000	0.28	2001	...	...		109 000	0.08	2001	203 000	0.16	2001	1 061 000	0.82	2001	1 077 000	0.83	2001
...	...		...	...		...	...		...	...		...	...		...	...	
41	0.05	2004	17	0.02	2004	41	0.05	2004	63	0.08	2004	10	0.01	2004	271	0.34	2004
99	0.03	2004	9	0.00	2004	124	0.03	2004	554	0.15	2004	957	0.25	2004	987	0.26	2004
2	0.11	2001	...	...		...	...		...	...		...	...		...	...	
2 101	0.53	2000	1 266	0.32	2000	5 071	1.29	2000	...	...		7 379	1.88	2000	18 406	4.68	2000
1 015	0.06	2004	155	0.01	2004	...	...		1 165	0.07	2004	172	0.01	2004	2 107	0.12	2004
2 348	0.53	2003	...	...		...	...		...	...		...	...		...	...	
...	...		...	...		...	...		...	...		...	...		...	...	
144	0.18	2002	...	...		...	...		...	...		...	...		...	...	
5 610	0.55	2003	...	...		...	...		...	...		...	...		...	...	
13 497	0.60	2003	2 685	0.12	2003	...	...		950	0.04	2003	67 957	3.00	2003	...	...	
1 200	0.02	2004	...	...		...	...		512	0.01	2004	1 042	0.02	2004	15 013	0.28	2004
2 638	0.49	2002	...	...		...	...		...	...		...	...		...	...	
18	0.03	2004	...	...		23	0.03	2004	84	0.12	2004	159	0.22	2004	232	0.33	2004
...	...		...	...		...	...		...	...		...	...		...	...	
3 330	0.40	2000	...	...		...	...		...	...		...	...		...	...	
...	...		...	...		...	...		...	...		...	...		...	...	
7 119	0.10	2004	9 531	0.13	2004	...	...		20 011	0.27	2004	3 694	0.05	2004	5 167	0.07	2004
...	...		...	...		...	...		...	...		...	...		...	...	

Health systems

Figures have been computed by WHO to ensure comparability; thus they are not necessarily the official statistics of Member States, which may use alternative rigorous methods.

	Member State	WHO region	Human resources for health[a]											
			Physicians			Nurses			Midwives			Dentists		
			Number	Density per 1 000 population	Year	Number	Density per 1 000 population	Year	Number	Density per 1 000 population	Year	Number	Density per 1 000 population	Year
56	Equatorial Guinea	AFR	153	0.30	2004	218	0.43	2004	53	0.10	2004	15	0.03	2004
57	Eritrea	AFR	215	0.05	2004	2 365	0.55	2004	140	0.03	2004	16	0.00	2004
58	Estonia	EUR	6 118	4.48	2000	11 618	8.50	2000	469	0.34	2000	1 747	1.28	2000
59	Ethiopia	AFR	1 936	0.03	2003	14 270	0.20	2003	1 274	0.02	2003	93	0.00	2003
60	Fiji	WPR	271	0.34	1999	1 576	1.96	1999	...	...		32	0.04	1999
61	Finland	EUR	16 446	3.16	2002	74 450	14.33	2002	3 952	0.76	2002	6 674	1.28	2002
62	France	EUR	203 487	3.37	2004	437 525	7.24	2004	15 684	0.26	2003	40 904	0.68	2004
63	Gabon	AFR	395	0.29	2004	6 275	4.64	2004	503	0.37	2004	66	0.05	2004
64	Gambia	AFR	156	0.11	2003	1 618	1.13	2003	263	0.18	2003	43	0.03	2003
65	Georgia	EUR	20 962	4.09	2003	17 807	3.47	2003	1 495	0.29	2003	1 438	0.28	2003
66	Germany	EUR	277 885	3.37	2003	801 677	9.72	2003	8 559	0.10	2002	64 609	0.78	2003
67	Ghana	AFR	3 240	0.15	2004	15 797	0.74	2004	3 910	0.18	2004	393	0.02	2004
68	Greece	EUR	47 944	4.38	2001	42 129	3.86	2000	1 916	0.18	2001	12 394	1.13	2001
69	Grenada	AMR	41	0.50	1997	303	3.70	1997	...	...		7	0.09	1997
70	Guatemala	AMR	9 965	0.90	1999	44 986	4.05	1999	...	...		2 046	0.18	1999
71	Guinea	AFR	987	0.11	2004	4 061	0.47	2004	347	0.04	2004	60	0.01	2004
72	Guinea-Bissau	AFR	188	0.12	2004	912	0.59	2004	160	0.10	2004	22	0.01	2004
73	Guyana	AMR	366	0.48	2000	1 738	2.29	2000	...	...		30	0.04	2000
74	Haiti	AMR	1 949	0.25	1998	834	0.11	1998	...	...		94	0.01	1998
75	Honduras	AMR	3 676	0.57	2000	8 333	1.29	2000	195	0.03	2000	1 371	0.21	2000
76	Hungary	EUR	32 877	3.33	2003	87 381	8.85	2003	2 032	0.21	2003	5 364	0.54	2003
77	Iceland	EUR	1 056	3.62	2004	3 954	13.63	2003	200	0.69	2003	283	1.00	2000
78	India	SEAR	645 825	0.60	2004	865 135	0.80	2004	506 924	0.47	2004	61 424	0.06	2004
79	Indonesia	SEAR	29 499	0.13	2003	125 621	0.57	2003	54 338	0.25	2003	7 093	0.03	2003
80	Iran (Islamic Republic of)	EMR	60 791	0.87	2004	83 175	1.19	2004	13 087	0.19	2004	13 135	0.19	2004
81	Iraq	EMR	17 022	0.66	2004	32 304	1.25	2004	1 701	0.07	2004	11 489	0.44	2004
82	Ireland	EUR	11 141	2.79	2004	60 774	15.20	2004	16 486	4.27	2001	2 237	0.56	2004
83	Israel	EUR	24 577	3.82	2003	40 280	6.26	2003	1 202	0.19	2003	7 510	1.17	2003
84	Italy	EUR	241 000	4.20	2004	312 377	5.44	2003	...	...		33 000	0.58	2004
85	Jamaica	AMR	2 253	0.85	2003	4 374	1.65	2003	...	...		212	0.08	2003
86	Japan	WPR	251 889	1.98	2002	993 628	7.79	2002	24 511	0.19	2000	90 510	0.71	2002
87	Jordan	EMR	11 398	2.03	2004	16 527	2.94	2004	1 669	0.30	2004	7 270	1.29	2004
88	Kazakhstan	EUR	54 613	3.54	2003	92 773	6.01	2003	8 018	0.52	2003	5 215	0.34	2003
89	Kenya	AFR	4 506	0.14	2002	37 113	1.18	2002	...	...		1 340	0.04	2002
90	Kiribati	WPR	24	0.30	1998	191	2.36	1998	...	...		4	0.05	1998
91	Kuwait	EMR	3 589	1.53	2001	9 197	3.91	2001	...	...		673	0.29	2001
92	Kyrgyzstan	EUR	12 902	2.51	2003	31 557	6.14	2003	2 663	0.52	2003	992	0.19	2003
93	Lao People's Democratic Republic	WPR	...	...		...	...		...	...		...	...	
94	Latvia	EUR	6 940	3.01	2003	12 150	5.27	2003	482	0.21	2003	1 287	0.56	2003
95	Lebanon	EMR	11 505	3.25	2001	4 157	1.18	2001	...	...		4 283	1.21	2001
96	Lesotho	AFR	89	0.05	2003	1 123	0.62	2003	...	...		16	0.01	2003
97	Liberia	AFR	103	0.03	2004	589	0.17	2004	446	0.13	2004	13	0.00	2004
98	Libyan Arab Jamahiriya	EMR	6 371	1.29	1997	17 779	3.60	1997	...	...		693	0.14	1997
99	Lithuania	EUR	13 682	3.97	2003	26 229	7.62	2003	1 132	0.33	2003	2 372	0.69	2003
100	Luxembourg	EUR	1 206	2.66	2003	4 151	9.16	2003	114	0.25	2003	323	0.71	2003
101	Madagascar	AFR	5 201	0.29	2004	3 585	0.20	2004	2 076	0.12	2004	410	0.02	2004
102	Malawi	AFR	266	0.02	2004	7 264	0.59	2004	...	...		...	...	
103	Malaysia	WPR	16 146	0.70	2000	31 129	1.35	2000	7 711	0.34	2000	2 144	0.09	2000
104	Maldives	SEAR	302	0.92	2004	886	2.70	2004	...	...		14	0.04	2004
105	Mali	AFR	1 053	0.08	2004	5 986	0.45	2004	2 352	0.18	2004	84	0.01	2004
106	Malta	EUR	1 254	3.18	2003	2 298	5.83	2003	125	0.32	2003	167	0.42	2003
107	Marshall Islands	WPR	24	0.47	2000	152	2.98	2000	...	...		4	0.08	2000
108	Mauritania	AFR	313	0.11	2004	1 658	0.56	2004	235	0.08	2004	64	0.02	2004
109	Mauritius	AFR	1 303	1.06	2004	4 438	3.60	2004	166	0.13	2004	233	0.19	2004
110	Mexico	AMR	195 897	1.98	2000	88 678	0.90	2000	...	...		78 281	0.79	2000

WORLD HEALTH STATISTICS 2007

Human resources for health[a]																				
Pharmacists			Public and environmental health workers			Community health workers			Laboratory health workers			Other health workers			Health management and support workers		
Number	Density per 1 000 population	Year	Number	Density per 1 000 population	Year	Number	Density per 1 000 population	Year	Number	Density per 1 000 population	Year	Number	Density per 1 000 population	Year	Number	Density per 1 000 population	Year
121	0.24	2004	18	0.04	2004	1 275	2.51	2004	84	0.17	2004	...	...		74	0.15	2004
107	0.02	2004	88	0.02	2004	...	...		248	0.06	2004	56	0.01	2004	765	0.18	2004
580	0.42	2000	115	0.08	2000	5 242	3.83	2000	...	...		597	0.44	2000	10 859	7.94	2000
1 343	0.02	2003	1 347	0.02	2003	18 652	0.26	2003	2 703	0.04	2003	7 354	0.10	2003	...	...	
59	0.07	1999	...	...		...	...		...	...		...	...		...	...	
5 829	1.12	2002	...	...		...	...		10 119	1.95	2002	19 202	3.69	2002	...	...	
63 909	1.06	2003	...	...		...	...		...	...		...	...		...	...	
63	0.05	2004	150	0.11	2004	...	...		276	0.20	2004	197	0.15	2004	144	0.11	2004
48	0.03	2003	33	0.02	2003	968	0.68	2003	99	0.07	2003	3	0.00	2003	391	0.27	2003
352	0.07	2003	...	...		...	...		...	...		...	...		...	...	
47 956	0.58	2003	...	...		...	...		...	...		...	...		...	...	
1 388	0.06	2004	...	...		...	...		899	0.04	2004	7 132	0.33	2004	19 151	0.90	2004
8 977	0.82	2000	...	...		...	...		...	...		...	...		...	...	
...	...		...	...		...	...		...	...		...	...		...	...	
...	...		...	...		...	...		...	...		...	...		...	...	
530	0.06	2004	135	0.02	2004	93	0.01	2004	268	0.03	2004	430	0.05	2004	511	0.06	2004
40	0.03	2004	13	0.01	2004	4 486	2.92	2004	230	0.15	2004	61	0.04	2004	38	0.02	2004
...	...		...	...		...	...		...	...		...	...		...	...	
...	...		...	...		...	...		...	...		...	...		...	...	
926	0.14	2000	215	0.03	2000	...	...		...	...		2 936	0.45	2000	...	...	
5 125	0.52	2003	...	...		...	...		...	...		...	...		...	...	
374	1.30	2002	...	...		...	...		...	...		...	...		...	...	
592 577	0.56	2003	...	...		50 393	0.05	2004	...	...		1 101 485	1.03	2003	...	...	
7 580	0.03	2003	6 493	0.03	2003	...	0.00	2003	8 882	0.04	2003	20 981	0.10	2003	228 095	1.04	2003
14 140	0.20	2004	10 004	0.14	2004	25 242	0.36	2004	20 049	0.29	2004	84 207	1.21	2004	72 905	1.04	2004
13 775	0.53	2004	2 601	0.10	2004	1 968	0.08	2004	12 184	0.47	2004	20 340	0.79	2004	34 273	1.33	2004
3 898	0.97	2004	...	...		...	...		...	...		...	...		...	...	
4 480	0.70	2003	...	...		...	...		...	...		...	...		...	...	
66 119	1.15	2003	...	...		...	...		...	...		...	...		...	...	
...	...		...	...		...	...		...	...		...	...		...	...	
154 428	1.21	2002	...	...		...	...		...	...		...	...		...	...	
17 654	3.14	2004	1 412	0.25	2004	1 000	0.18	2004	5 630	1.00	2004	6 569	1.17	2004	17 668	3.15	2004
10 390	0.67	2003	...	...		...	...		...	...		...	...		...	...	
3 094	0.10	2004	6 496	0.20	2004	...	...		7 000	0.22	2004	5 610	0.17	2004	1 797	0.06	2004
4	0.05	1998	...	...		...	...		...	...		...	...		...	...	
722	0.31	2001	...	...		...	...		...	...		...	...		...	...	
158	0.03	2003	...	...		...	...		...	...		...	...		...	...	
...	...		...	...		...	...		...	...		...	...		...	...	
...	...		...	...		...	...		...	...		...	...		...	...	
3 359	0.95	2001	...	...		...	...		...	...		...	...		...	...	
62	0.03	2003	55	0.03	2003	...	...		146	0.08	2003	35	0.02	2003	6	0.00	2003
35	0.01	2004	150	0.04	2004	142	0.04	2004	218	0.06	2004	540	0.15	2004	518	0.15	2004
1 225	0.25	1997	...	...		...	...		...	...		...	...		...	...	
2 390	0.69	2003	...	...		...	...		...	...		...	...		...	...	
371	0.82	2003	...	...		...	...		...	...		...	...		...	...	
175	0.01	2004	130	0.01	2004	385	0.02	2004	172	0.01	2004	530	0.03	2004	6 036	0.34	2004
...	...		26	0.00	2004	...	...		46	0.00	2004	707	0.06	2004	...	...	
2 333	0.10	2000	...	...		...	...		...	...		...	...		...	...	
241	0.73	2004	...	...		919	2.80	2004	168	0.51	2004	14	0.04	2004	...	...	
351	0.03	2004	231	0.02	2004	68	0.01	2004	264	0.02	2004	377	0.03	2004	652	0.05	2004
800	2.03	2003	...	...		...	...		...	...		...	...		...	...	
2	0.04	2000	...	...		...	...		...	...		...	...		...	...	
81	0.03	2004	...	...		429	0.14	2004	106	0.04	2004	48	0.02	2004	1 056	0.35	2004
1 428	1.16	2004	238	0.19	2004	236	0.19	2004	324	0.26	2004	145	0.12	2004	2 027	1.64	2004
3 189	0.03	2000	...	...		...	...		45 482	0.46	2000	236 861	2.39	2000	412 319	4.17	2000

Health systems

Figures have been computed by WHO to ensure comparability; thus they are not necessarily the official statistics of Member States, which may use alternative rigorous methods.

	Member State	WHO region	Physicians			Nurses			Midwives			Dentists		
			Number	Density per 1 000 population	Year	Number	Density per 1 000 population	Year	Number	Density per 1 000 population	Year	Number	Density per 1 000 population	Year
111	Micronesia (Federated States of)	WPR	64	0.60	2000	410	3.83	2000	7	0.07	2000	14	0.13	2000
112	Monaco	EUR	...	...		...	...		...	...		...	...	
113	Mongolia	WPR	6 732	2.63	2002	8 214	3.21	2002	612	0.24	2002	337	0.13	2002
114	Montenegro	EUR	...	...		...	...		...	...		...	...	
115	Morocco	EMR	15 991	0.51	2004	22 250	0.72	2004	2 078	0.07	2004	3 091	0.10	2004
116	Mozambique	AFR	514	0.03	2004	3 947	0.21	2004	2 236	0.12	2004	159	0.01	2004
117	Myanmar	SEAR	17 791	0.36	2004	9 899	0.20	2004	39 442	0.79	2004	1 396	0.03	2004
118	Namibia	AFR	598	0.30	2004	6 145	3.06	2004	...	...		113	0.06	2004
119	Nauru	WPR	...	...		...	...		...	...		...	...	
120	Nepal	SEAR	5 384	0.21	2004	5 664	0.22	2004	6 161	0.24	2004	359	0.01	2004
121	Netherlands	EUR	50 854	3.15	2003	221 783	13.73	2003	1 940	0.12	2003	7 759	0.48	2003
122	New Zealand	WPR	9 027	2.37	2001	31 128	8.16	2001	2 121	0.56	2001	2 586	0.68	2001
123	Nicaragua	AMR	2 045	0.37	2003	5 862	1.07	2003	...	...		243	0.04	2003
124	Niger	AFR	296	0.02	2004	2 421	0.20	2004	397	0.03	2004	15	0.00	2004
125	Nigeria	AFR	34 923	0.28	2003	127 580	1.03	2003	82 726	0.67	2003	2 482	0.02	2003
126	Niue	WPR	...	...		...	...		...	...		...	...	
127	Norway	EUR	14 200	3.13	2003	67 274	14.84	2003	2 243	0.49	2003	3 733	0.82	2003
128	Oman	EMR	3 871	1.32	2004	10 273	3.50	2004	16	0.01	2004	544	0.19	2004
129	Pakistan	EMR	116 298	0.74	2004	48 446	0.31	2004	23 318	0.15	2004	7 862	0.05	2004
130	Palau	WPR	20	1.11	1998	26	1.44	1998	1	0.06	1998	2	0.11	1998
131	Panama	AMR	4 431	1.50	2000	8 158	2.77	2000	...	...		2 231	0.76	2000
132	Papua New Guinea	WPR	275	0.05	2000	2 841	0.53	2000	...	...		90	0.02	2000
133	Paraguay	AMR	6 355	1.11	2002	9 727	1.69	2002	534	0.09	2002	3 182	0.55	2002
134	Peru	AMR	29 799	1.17	1999	17 108	0.67	1999	...	...		2 809	0.11	1999
135	Philippines	WPR	44 287	0.58	2000	127 595	1.69	2000	33 963	0.45	2000	8 564	0.11	2000
136	Poland	EUR	95 272	2.47	2003	188 898	4.90	2003	21 997	0.57	2002	11 451	0.30	2003
137	Portugal	EUR	34 440	3.42	2003	43 860	4.36	2003	824	0.08	2000	5 510	0.55	2003
138	Qatar	EMR	1 310	2.22	2001	2 917	4.94	2001	...	...		220	0.37	2001
139	Republic of Korea	WPR	75 045	1.57	2003	83 333	1.75	2003	8 728	0.19	2000	16 033	0.34	2003
140	Republic of Moldova	EUR	11 246	2.64	2003	25 848	6.06	2003	991	0.23	2003	1 403	0.33	2003
141	Romania	EUR	42 538	1.90	2003	86 802	3.89	2003	5 571	0.25	2003	4 919	0.22	2003
142	Russian Federation	EUR	609 043	4.25	2003	1 153 683	8.05	2003	67 403	0.47	2003	45 972	0.32	2003
143	Rwanda	AFR	432	0.05	2004	3 570	0.42	2004	77	0.01	2004	21	0.00	2004
144	Saint Kitts and Nevis	AMR	51	1.19	1997	216	5.02	1997	...	...		8	0.19	1997
145	Saint Lucia	AMR	749	5.17	1999	331	2.28	1999	...	...		9	0.06	1999
146	Saint Vincent and the Grenadines	AMR	101	0.87	1997	276	2.38	1997	...	...		6	0.05	1997
147	Samoa	WPR	120	0.70	1999	346	2.02	1999	3	0.02	1999	30	0.18	1999
148	San Marino	EUR	...	...		...	...		...	...		...	...	
149	Sao Tome and Principe	AFR	81	0.49	2004	256	1.55	2004	52	0.32	2004	11	0.07	2004
150	Saudi Arabia	EMR	34 261	1.37	2004	74 114	2.97	2004	...	...		4 235	0.17	2004
151	Senegal	AFR	594	0.06	2004	2 606	0.25	2004	681	0.07	2004	97	0.01	2004
152	Serbia	EUR	...	...		...	...		...	...		...	...	
153	Seychelles	AFR	121	1.51	2004	634	7.93	2004	...	...		94	1.18	2004
154	Sierra Leone	AFR	162	0.03	2004	1 211	0.23	2004	1 299	0.25	2004	5	0.00	2004
155	Singapore	WPR	5 747	1.40	2001	17 398	4.24	2001	...	...		1 087	0.26	2001
156	Slovakia	EUR	17 172	3.18	2003	36 569	6.77	2003	1 456	0.27	2003	2 364	0.44	2003
157	Slovenia	EUR	4 475	2.25	2002	14 327	7.21	2002	654	0.33	2001	1 199	0.60	2002
158	Solomon Islands	WPR	54	0.13	1999	338	0.80	1999	23	0.05	1999	26	0.06	1999
159	Somalia	EMR	310	0.04	1997	1 486	0.19	1997	...	...		15	0.00	1997
160	South Africa	AFR	34 829	0.77	2004	184 459	4.08	2004	...	...		5 995	0.13	2004
161	Spain	EUR	135 300	3.30	2003	315 200	7.68	2003	6 291	0.15	2001	20 005	0.49	2003
162	Sri Lanka	SEAR	10 479	0.55	2004	23 030	1.20	2004	10 401	0.54	2004	1 245	0.06	2004
163	Sudan	EMR	7 552	0.22	2004	17 656	0.51	2004	13 840	0.40	2004	1 082	0.03	2004
164	Suriname	AMR	191	0.45	2000	688	1.62	2000	...	...		4	0.01	2000
165	Swaziland	AFR	171	0.16	2004	4 590	4.24	2004	2 238	2.07	2004	32	0.03	2004

World Health Statistics 2007

Pharmacists			Public and environmental health workers			Community health workers			Laboratory health workers			Other health workers			Health management and support workers		
Number	Density per 1 000 population	Year	Number	Density per 1 000 population	Year	Number	Density per 1 000 population	Year	Number	Density per 1 000 population	Year	Number	Density per 1 000 population	Year	Number	Density per 1 000 population	Year
...	...		...	...		...	...		...	...		...	...		...	...	
1 093	0.43	2002	85	0.03	2002	3 758	1.47	2002	...	...		3 389	1.32	2002	...	...	
7 366	0.24	2004	737	0.02	2004	...	...		1 470	0.05	2004	1 123	0.04	2004	6 300	0.20	2004
618	0.03	2004	564	0.03	2004	...	...		941	0.05	2004	1 659	0.09	2004	9 491	0.49	2004
127	0.00	2004	1 757	0.04	2004	49 531	0.99	2004	2 241	0.04	2004	2 077	0.04	2004	49 661	0.99	2004
288	0.14	2004	240	0.12	2004	...	...		481	0.24	2004	597	0.30	2004	7 782	3.87	2004
...	...		...	...		...	...		...	...		...	...		...	...	
358	0.01	2004	172	0.01	2004	16 206	0.63	2004	3 209	0.12	2004	1 892	0.07	2004	...	...	
3 134	0.19	2003	...	...		...	...		...	...		...	...		...	...	
3 495	0.92	2001	...	...		30 987	8.12	2001	3 696	0.97	2001	17 013	4.46	2001	...	...	
...	...		...	...		...	...		...	...		...	...		...	...	
20	0.00	2004	268	0.02	2004	...	...		294	0.02	2004	485	0.04	2004	241	0.02	2004
6 344	0.05	2004	...	...		115 761	0.91	2004	690	0.01	2004	1 220	0.01	2004	...	...	
...	...		...	...		...	...		...	...		...	...		...	...	
1 675	0.37	2003	...	...		...	...		...	...		...	...		...	...	
1 551	0.53	2004	173	0.06	2004	...	...		1 049	0.36	2004	1 256	0.43	2004	3 898	1.33	2004
8 102	0.05	2004	106	0.00	2004	65 999	0.42	2004	9 744	0.06	2004	19 082	0.12	2004	203 337	1.29	2004
1	0.06	1998	...	...		...	...		...	...		...	...		...	...	
2 526	0.86	2000	948	0.32	2000	1 359	0.46	2000	...	...		870	0.29	2000	6 862	2.33	2000
...	...		...	...		...	...		...	...		...	...		...	...	
1 868	0.33	2002	133	0.02	2002	6 598	1.15	2002	...	...		2 235	0.39	2002	...	...	
...	...		...	...		...	...		...	...		...	...		...	...	
2 482	0.03	2000	...	...		...	...		...	...		90 788	1.20	2000	...	...	
25 397	0.66	2003	...	...		...	...		...	...		...	...		...	...	
9 543	0.95	2003	...	...		...	...		...	...		...	...		...	...	
530	0.90	2001	...	...		...	...		...	...		...	...		...	...	
50 623	1.08	2000	...	...		...	...		...	...		...	...		...	...	
2 061	0.48	2003	...	...		...	...		...	...		...	...		...	...	
1 275	0.06	2003	...	...		...	...		...	...		...	...		...	...	
11 404	0.08	2003	72 515	0.50	2000	435 093	2.99	2000	...	...		670 768	4.61	2000	...	...	
278	0.03	2004	101	0.01	2004	12 557	1.48	2004	39	0.00	2004	490	0.06	2004	862	0.10	2004
...	...		...	...		...	...		...	...		...	...		...	...	
...	...		...	...		...	...		...	...		...	...		...	...	
...	...		...	...		...	...		...	...		...	...		...	...	
5	0.03	1999	...	...		...	...		...	...		...	...		...	...	
...	...		...	...		...	...		...	...		...	...		...	...	
24	0.15	2004	19	0.12	2004	374	2.27	2004	51	0.31	2004	291	1.76	2004	288	1.75	2004
5 485	0.22	2004	...	...		...	...		...	...		39 073	1.57	2004	...	...	
85	0.01	2004	705	0.07	2004	...	...		66	0.01	2004	704	0.07	2004	564	0.05	2004
...	...		...	...		...	...		...	...		...	...		...	...	
61	0.76	2004	77	0.96	2004	...	...		59	0.74	2004	35	0.44	2004	...	...	
340	0.07	2004	136	0.03	2004	558	0.11	2004	...	...		4	0.00	2004	6	0.00	2004
1 141	0.28	2001	...	...		...	...		...	...		...	...		...	...	
2 783	0.52	2003	...	...		...	...		...	...		...	...		...	...	
790	0.40	2002	...	...		...	...		...	...		...	...		...	...	
28	0.07	1999	...	...		...	...		...	...		...	...		...	...	
8	0.00	1997	...	...		...	...		...	...		...	...		...	...	
12 521	0.28	2004	2 529	0.06	2004	14 306	0.32	2004	2 002	0.04	2004	40 492	0.90	2004	22 859	0.51	2004
35 800	0.87	2003	...	...		...	...		...	...		...	...		...	...	
1 066	0.06	2004	1 541	0.08	2004	...	...		1 252	0.07	2004	1 546	0.08	2004	112	0.01	2004
3 558	0.10	2004	2 897	0.08	2004	5 797	0.17	2004	3 115	0.09	2004	8 667	0.25	2004	35 374	1.03	2004
...	...		...	...		...	...		...	...		...	...		...	...	
70	0.06	2004	110	0.10	2004	4 700	4.34	2004	77	0.07	2004	616	0.57	2004	310	0.29	2004

Health systems

Figures have been computed by WHO to ensure comparability; thus they are not necessarily the official statistics of Member States, which may use alternative rigorous methods.

	Member State	WHO region	Physicians			Nurses			Midwives			Dentists		
			Number	Density per 1 000 population	Year	Number	Density per 1 000 population	Year	Number	Density per 1 000 population	Year	Number	Density per 1 000 population	Year
166	Sweden	EUR	29 122	3.28	2002	90 758	10.24	2002	6 247	0.70	2002	7 270	0.82	2002
167	Switzerland	EUR	25 921	3.61	2002	77 120	10.75	2000	2 033	0.28	2000	3 598	0.50	2003
168	Syrian Arab Republic	EMR	23 742	1.40	2001	32 938	1.94	2001	...	...		12 206	0.72	2001
169	Tajikistan	EUR	12 697	2.03	2003	28 586	4.58	2003	3 780	0.61	2003	945	0.15	2003
170	Thailand	SEAR	22 435	0.37	2000	171 605	2.82	2000	872	0.01	2000	10 459	0.17	2000
171	The former Yugoslav Republic of Macedonia	EUR	4 459	2.19	2001	10 553	5.19	2001	1 456	0.72	2001	1 125	0.55	2001
172	Timor-Leste	SEAR	79	0.10	2004	1 467	1.79	2004	328	0.40	2004	45	0.05	2004
173	Togo	AFR	225	0.04	2004	1 667	0.33	2004	270	0.05	2004	19	0.00	2004
174	Tonga	WPR	35	0.34	2001	322	3.16	2001	19	0.19	2001	33	0.32	2001
175	Trinidad and Tobago	AMR	1 004	0.79	1997	3 653	2.87	1997	...	...		107	0.08	1997
176	Tunisia	EMR	13 330	1.34	2004	25 654	2.58	2004	2 883	0.29	2004	2 452	0.25	2004
177	Turkey	EUR	96 000	1.35	2003	121 000	1.70	2003	...	...		17 200	0.24	2003
178	Turkmenistan	EUR	20 032	4.18	2002	43 359	9.04	2002	...	...		876	0.18	2002
179	Tuvalu	WPR	6	0.55	2002	29	2.64	2002	10	0.91	2002	2	0.18	2002
180	Uganda	AFR	2 209	0.08	2004	14 805	0.55	2004	4 164	0.16	2004	363	0.01	2004
181	Ukraine	EUR	143 202	2.95	2003	369 755	7.62	2003	24 496	0.50	2003	19 354	0.40	2003
182	United Arab Emirates	EMR	5 825	2.02	2001	12 045	4.18	2001	...	...		954	0.33	2001
183	United Kingdom	EUR	133 641	2.30	1997	704 332	12.12	1997	36 399	0.63	1997	58 729	1.01	1997
184	United Republic of Tanzania	AFR	822	0.02	2002	10 729	0.30	2002	2 563	0.07	2002	267	0.01	2002
185	United States of America	AMR	730 801	2.56	2000	2 669 603	9.37	2000	...	...		463 663	1.63	2000
186	Uruguay	AMR	12 384	3.65	2002	2 880	0.85	2002	...	...		3 936	1.16	2002
187	Uzbekistan	EUR	71 623	2.74	2003	256 183	9.82	2003	21 270	0.82	2003	3 606	0.14	2003
188	Vanuatu	WPR	20	0.11	1997	428	2.35	1997	...	...		...	...	
189	Venezuela (Bolivarian Republic of)	AMR	48 000	1.94	2001	15 020	0.66	1997	...	...		13 680	0.55	2001
190	Viet Nam	WPR	42 327	0.53	2001	44 539	0.56	2001	14 662	0.19	2001	...	...	
191	Yemen	EMR	6 739	0.33	2004	13 333	0.64	2004	413	0.02	2004	850	0.04	2004
192	Zambia	AFR	1 264	0.12	2004	16 990	1.56	2004	5 020	0.46	2004	491	0.04	2004
193	Zimbabwe	AFR	2 086	0.16	2004	9 357	0.72	2004	...	...		310	0.02	2004
194	The former state union of Serbia and Montenegro[b]	EUR	21 738	2.06	2002	48 875	4.64	2002	2 864	0.27	2002	3 792	0.36	2002

Region													
African Region	AFR	150 708	0.21		663 942	0.93		...	...		23 964	0.03	
Region of the Americas	AMR	1 624 583	1.94		4 063 609	4.88		...	...		880 636	1.05	
South-East Asia Region	SEAR	844 994	0.52		1 311 301	0.81		...	...		92 945	0.06	
European Region	EUR	2 810 063	3.20		6 529 455	7.43		...	...		450 624	0.52	
Eastern Mediterranean Region	EMR	383 426	0.74		577 161	1.11		...	...		81 953	0.16	
Western Pacific Region	WPR	1 869 216	1.10		2 891 839	1.70		...	...		279 779	0.17	
Global		7 682 990	1.23		16 037 307	2.56		...	...		1 809 901	0.29	

... Data not available or not applicable; AFR, African Region; AMR, Region of the Americas; SEAR, South-East Asia Region; EUR, European Region; EMR, Eastern Mediterranean Region; WPR, Western Pacific Region.

The global values for rates and ratios are weighted averages; for absolute numbers they are the sums of all WHO regions.

[a] Global Atlas of the Health Workforce [online database]. World Health Organization. (http://who.int/globalatlas/autologin/hrh_login.asp, accessed 1 March 2007).

[b] See footnote o to the table on Health status: mortality.

Human resources for health[a]																		
Pharmacists			Public and environmental health workers			Community health workers			Laboratory health workers			Other health workers			Health management and support workers		
Number	Density per 1 000 population	Year	Number	Density per 1 000 population	Year	Number	Density per 1 000 population	Year	Number	Density per 1 000 population	Year	Number	Density per 1 000 population	Year	Number	Density per 1 000 population	Year
5 885	0.66	2002	...	...		...	...		...	...		...	...		...	...	
4 322	0.60	2003	...	...		...	...		...	...		...	...		...	...	
8 862	0.52	2001	...	...		...	...		...	...		...	...		...	...	
680	0.11	2003	...	...		...	...		...	...		...	...		...	...	
15 480	0.25	2000	2 151	0.04	2000	39 780	0.65	2000	...	...		14 117	0.23	2000	117 384	1.93	2000
309	0.15	2001	...	...		...	...		...	...		...	...		...	...	
14	0.02	2004	22	0.03	2004	1 657	2.02	2004	36	0.04	2004	18	0.02	2004	184	0.22	2004
134	0.03	2004	289	0.06	2004	475	0.09	2004	528	0.11	2004	606	0.12	2004	1 335	0.27	2004
17	0.17	2001	...	...		...	...		...	...		...	...		...	...	
...	...		...	...		...	...		...	...		...	...		...	...	
2 909	0.29	2004	890	0.09	2004	...	...		3 936	0.40	2004	10 799	1.09	2004	15 955	1.61	2004
22 500	0.32	2003	...	...		...	...		...	...		...	...		...	...	
1 626	0.34	2002	...	...		...	...		...	...		7 846	1.64	2002	...	...	
1	0.09	2002	...	...		...	...		...	...		...	...		...	...	
688	0.03	2004	1 042	0.04	2004	...	...		1 702	0.06	2004	4 128	0.15	2004	6 344	0.24	2004
23 576	0.48	2001	...	...		...	...		...	...		...	...		...	...	
1 086	0.38	2001	...	...		...	...		...	...		...	...		...	...	
29 726	0.51	1997	14 439	0.25	1997	490 002	8.43	1997	20 035	0.34	1997	161 490	2.78	1997	741 664	12.77	1997
365	0.01	2002	1 831	0.05	2002	...	...		1 520	0.04	2002	29 722	0.82	2002	689	0.02	2002
249 642	0.88	2000	...	...		...	...		651 035	2.28	2000	4 138 567	14.52	2000	7 056 080	24.76	2000
...	...		...	...		...	...		...	...		...	...		...	...	
899	0.03	2003	...	...		...	...		...	...		...	...		...	...	
...	...		...	...		...	...		...	...		...	...		...	...	
...	...		...	...		...	...		...	...		...	...		...	...	
5 977	0.08	2001	...	...		...	...		...	...		...	...		...	...	
2 638	0.13	2004	792	0.04	2004	6 025	0.29	2004	4 709	0.23	2004	4 580	0.22	2004	10 902	0.53	2004
1 039	0.10	2004	1 027	0.09	2004	...	...		1 415	0.13	2004	3 330	0.30	2004	10 853	0.99	2004
883	0.07	2004	1 803	0.14	2004	581	0.04	2004	917	0.07	2004	743	0.06	2004	...	...	
1 980	0.19	2002	...	...		...	...		...	...		...	...		...	...	

Health systems

Figures have been computed by WHO to ensure comparability; thus they are not necessarily the official statistics of Member States, which may use alternative rigorous methods.

	Member State	WHO region	Health expenditure ratios						
			Total expenditure on health as % of gross domestic product[a]	General government expenditure on health as % of total expenditure on health[a,b]	Private expenditure on health as % of total expenditure on health[a,b]	General government expenditure on health as % of total government expenditure[a]	External resources for health as % of total expenditure on health[a]	Social security expenditure on health as % of general government expenditure on health[a]	Out-of-pocket expenditure as % of private expenditure on health[a]
			2004	2004	2004	2004	2004	2004	2004
1	Afghanistan	EMR	4.4[e]	16.9	83.1	2.3	6.1	0.0	97.7
2	Albania	EUR	6.7	44.1	55.9	10.0	2.4	24.8	99.8
3	Algeria	AFR	3.6	72.5	27.5	8.4	0.0	33.2	94.6
4	Andorra	EUR	7.1	69.2	30.8	33.4	0.0	89.1	70.7
5	Angola	AFR	1.9	79.4	20.6	4.4	9.1	0.0	100.0
6	Antigua and Barbuda	AMR	4.8	70.6	29.4	12.4	0.9	0.0	100.0
7	Argentina	AMR	9.6	45.3	54.7	15.1	0.2	56.8	48.7
8	Armenia	EUR	5.4	26.2	73.8	6.8	7.2	0.0	89.2
9	Australia	WPR	9.6	67.5	32.5	18.5	0.0	0.0	61.6
10	Austria	EUR	10.3	75.6	24.4	15.4	0.0	61.0	67.9
11	Azerbaijan	EUR	3.6	25.0	75.0	3.4	1.6	0.0	93.6
12	Bahamas	AMR	6.8	50.1	49.9	15.1	0.2	2.6	40.3
13	Bahrain	EMR	4.0	67.2	32.8	9.4	0.0	0.5	69.3
14	Bangladesh	SEAR	3.1	28.1	71.9	5.9	15.1	0.0	88.3
15	Barbados	AMR	7.1	63.5	36.5	12.3	2.0	0.0	78.6
16	Belarus	EUR	6.2	74.9	25.1	10.2	...	2.2	72.7
17	Belgium	EUR	9.7	71.1	28.9	14.1	0.0	83.2	83.5
18	Belize	AMR	5.1	53.8	46.2	6.5	5.3	17.4	100.0
19	Benin	AFR	4.9	51.2	48.8	9.8	10.2	...	99.9
20	Bhutan	SEAR	4.6	64.2	35.8	6.1	14.5	0.0	100.0
21	Bolivia	AMR	6.8	60.7	39.3	12.8	9.1	65.3	82.5
22	Bosnia and Herzegovina	EUR	8.3	49.4	50.6	9.8	1.3	95.4	100.0
23	Botswana	AFR	6.4	62.9	37.1	10.5	2.5	...	27.9
24	Brazil	AMR	8.8	54.1	45.9	14.2	0.0	0.0	64.2
25	Brunei Darussalam	WPR	3.2	79.7	20.3	4.8	...	...	100.0
26	Bulgaria	EUR	8.0	57.6	42.4	11.6	1.0	49.6	98.0
27	Burkina Faso	AFR	6.1	54.8	45.2	15.3	26.8	0.4	97.9
28	Burundi	AFR	3.2	26.2	73.8	2.3	17.6	...	100.0
29	Cambodia	WPR	6.7	25.8	74.2	11.4	28.5	0.0	85.4
30	Cameroon	AFR	5.2	28.0	72.0	10.5	5.3	0.0	94.5
31	Canada	AMR	9.8	69.8	30.2	17.1	0.0	2.1	49.4
32	Cape Verde	AFR	5.2	75.8	24.2	12.3	20.7	29.5	99.8
33	Central African Republic	AFR	4.1	36.8	63.2	10.9	47.7	...	95.4
34	Chad	AFR	4.2	36.9	63.1	9.5	7.0	...	95.8
35	Chile	AMR	6.1	47.0	53.0	13.1	0.1	33.3	45.9
36	China	WPR	4.7[f]	38.0[f]	62.0[f]	10.1[f]	0.1[f]	55.2[f]	86.5[f]
37	Colombia	AMR	7.8	86.0	14.0	20.9	0.1	59.6	49.0
38	Comoros	AFR	2.8	56.9	43.1	8.0	18.3	0.0	100.0
39	Congo	AFR	2.5	49.2	50.8	4.4	3.6	0.0	100.0
40	Cook Islands	WPR	3.5	87.4	12.6	8.4	20.3	0.0	100.0
41	Costa Rica	AMR	6.6	77.0	23.0	21.3	0.8	90.6	88.7
42	Côte d'Ivoire	AFR	3.8	23.8	76.2	4.6	5.0	...	88.7
43	Croatia	EUR	7.7	81.0	19.0	14.1	0.4	97.9	93.8
44	Cuba	AMR	6.3	87.8	12.2	11.2	0.3	0.0	74.5
45	Cyprus	EUR	5.8	44.3	55.7	5.9	0.0	0.0	93.4

World Health Statistics 2007

	Health expenditure aggregates				Coverage of vital registration of deaths[c]		Hospital beds[a]	
Private prepaid plans as % of private expenditure on health[a]	Per capita total expenditure on health at average exchange rate[a] (US$)	Per capita total expenditure on health at international dollar rate[a]	Per capita government expenditure on health at average exchange rate[a] (US$)	Per capita government expenditure on health at international dollar rate[a]				
2004	2004	2004	2004	2004	(%)	Year	per 10 000 population	Year
0.0	14	19	2	3	<25	2002	4	
0.0	157	339	69	149	94	2003	30	2005
5.2	94	167	68	121	76	2000	17	2004
26.8	2 453	3 546	1 697	2 453	46	2000	27	2005
0.0	26	38	20	30	<25	2002	...	
...	485	516	343	365	...		24	2005
45.6	383	1 274	174	578	100	2003	41	2000
0.2	63	226	17	59	78	2003	45	2005
20.4	3 123	3 123	2 107	2 107	100	2002	40	2002
33.6	3 683	3 418	2 783	2 582	100	2004	77	2005
0.4	37	138	9	35	72	2002	82	2005
58.6	1 211	1 349	607	676	88	2000	34	2004
12.8	620	871	417	586	90	2001	28	2005
0.1	14	64	4	18	<25	2002	3	2001
21.4	745	1 151	473	731	100	2000	73	2004
0.1	147	427	110	319	98	2003	111	2005
12.0	3 363	3 133	2 392	2 228	100	1997	53	2005
...	201	339	108	182	96	2001	13	2004
0.1	24	40	12	21	<25	2002	5	2005
0.0	15	93	10	60	<25	2002	16	2001
8.8	66	186	40	113	<25	2002	10	2004
...	198	603	98	298	88	1999	30	2005
19.8	329	504	207	317	22	1998	22	2003
35.8	290	1 520	157	822	79	2000	26	2002
...	473	621	377	495	100	2000	27	2002
0.2	251	671	144	386	100	2003	64	2005
1.4	24	77	13	42	<25	2002	...	
...	3	16	1	4	<25	2002	7	2006
0.0	24	140	6	36	<25	2002	6	2001
...	51	83	14	23	<25	2002	...	
42.3	3 038	3 173	2 121	2 215	100	2002	36	2003
0.2	98	225	74	171	...		...	
...	13	54	5	20	<25	2002	...	
0.5	20	42	7	15	<25	2002	4	2005
54.0	359	720	169	338	98	2002	24	2004
5.5[f]	70[f]	277[f]	27[f]	105[f]	8	2000	22	2003
51.0	168	570	145	490	79	1999	12	2004
0.0	13	25	8	14	<25	2002	22	2006
...	28	30	14	15	<25	2002	...	
0.0	335	435	293	380	>75	2001	40	2004
2.1	290	592	223	456	79	2002	14	2004
11.3	33	64	8	15	<25	2002	...	
6.2	609	917	494	743	99	2004	55	2005
0.0	230	229	202	201	100	2003	49	2005
5.4	1 109	1 128	491	499	83	2003	34	2005

Health systems

Figures have been computed by WHO to ensure comparability; thus they are not necessarily the official statistics of Member States, which may use alternative rigorous methods.

	Member State	WHO region	Health expenditure ratios						
			Total expenditure on health as % of gross domestic product[a]	General government expenditure on health as % of total expenditure on health[a,b]	Private expenditure on health as % of total expenditure on health[a,b]	General government expenditure on health as % of total government expenditure[a]	External resources for health as % of total expenditure on health[a]	Social security expenditure on health as % of general government expenditure on health[a]	Out-of-pocket expenditure as % of private expenditure on health[a]
			2004	2004	2004	2004	2004	2004	2004
46	Czech Republic	EUR	7.3	89.2	10.8	14.6	0.0	89.2	95.5
47	Democratic People's Republic of Korea	SEAR	3.5	85.6	14.4	6.0	53.6	0.0	100.0
48	Democratic Republic of the Congo	AFR	4.0	28.1	71.9	7.3	19.1	0.0	100.0
49	Denmark	EUR	8.6	82.3	17.7	12.8	0.0	0.0	81.3
50	Djibouti	EMR	6.3	69.2	30.8	11.5	34.0	9.8	98.6
51	Dominica	AMR	5.9	71.3	28.7	11.9	3.0	0.0	100.0
52	Dominican Republic	AMR	6.0	31.6	68.4	10.3	1.5	16.2	73.1
53	Ecuador	AMR	5.5	40.7	59.3	7.6	0.8	39.2	85.4
54	Egypt	EMR	6.1	38.2	61.8	7.9	0.9	26.7	94.3
55	El Salvador	AMR	7.9	44.4	55.6	20.6	1.2	41.7	94.2
56	Equatorial Guinea	AFR	1.6	77.1	22.9	7.0	3.8	0.0	75.1
57	Eritrea	AFR	4.5	39.2	60.8	4.2	59.6	0.0	100.0
58	Estonia	EUR	5.3	76.0	24.0	11.5	0.5	86.5	88.8
59	Ethiopia	AFR	5.3	51.5	48.5	9.4	35.2	0.4	78.3
60	Fiji	WPR	4.6	62.3	37.7	9.1	9.6	0.0	100.0
61	Finland	EUR	7.4	77.2	22.8	11.3	0.0	21.9	80.8
62	France	EUR	10.5	78.4	21.6	15.4	0.0	95.7	34.9
63	Gabon	AFR	4.5	68.8	31.2	13.9	1.3	1.7	100.0
64	Gambia	AFR	6.8	27.1	72.9	5.9	23.0	0.0	68.2
65	Georgia	EUR	5.3	27.4	72.6	7.7	9.8	58.7	87.2
66	Germany	EUR	10.6	76.9	23.1	17.3	0.0	87.0	57.5
67	Ghana	AFR	6.7	42.2	57.8	8.4	29.9	...	78.2
68	Greece	EUR	7.9[g]	52.8	47.2	10.7	...	56.0	95.7
69	Grenada	AMR	6.9	72.8	27.2	11.1	1.5	0.0	100.0
70	Guatemala	AMR	5.7	41.0	59.0	18.8	2.3	49.4	90.5
71	Guinea	AFR	5.3	13.2	86.8	4.5	9.5	1.6	99.5
72	Guinea-Bissau	AFR	4.8	27.3	72.7	3.5	31.6	3.5	90.0
73	Guyana	AMR	5.3	83.5	16.5	10.0	8.2	0.0	100.0
74	Haiti	AMR	7.6	38.5	61.5	23.9	14.2	0.0	69.6
75	Honduras	AMR	7.2	54.9	45.1	16.7	8.7	14.2	84.3
76	Hungary	EUR	7.9	71.6	28.4	11.6	0.4	85.3	88.0
77	Iceland	EUR	9.9	83.4	16.6	18.1	0.0	37.0	100.0
78	India	SEAR	5.0	17.3	82.7	2.9	0.5	5.6	93.8
79	Indonesia	SEAR	2.8	34.2	65.8	5.0	1.3	10.8	74.7
80	Iran (Islamic Republic of)	EMR	6.6	47.8	52.2	10.9	0.2[c]	38.4	94.8
81	Iraq	EMR	5.3[h]	78.5[h]	21.5[h]	3.4[h]	2.5[h]	...	100.0[h]
82	Ireland	EUR	7.2	79.5	20.5	16.8	0.0	0.8	65.9
83	Israel	EUR	8.7	70.0	30.0	11.8	3.2	58.3	75.0
84	Italy	EUR	8.7	75.1	24.9	13.7	0.0	0.1	84.4
85	Jamaica	AMR	5.2	54.3	45.7	4.7	1.4	0.0	63.6
86	Japan	WPR	7.8	81.3	18.7	17.2	0.0	80.0	94.9
87	Jordan	EMR	9.8[i]	48.4[i]	51.6[i]	9.6[i]	7.1[i]	0.5[i]	73.8[i]
88	Kazakhstan	EUR	3.8	59.8	40.2	10.2	0.9	0.0	100.0
89	Kenya	AFR	4.1	42.7	57.3	8.2	18.3	8.4	81.9
90	Kiribati	WPR	13.7	93.0	7.0	9.3	27.9	0.0	100.0

World Health Statistics 2007

	Health expenditure aggregates				Coverage of vital registration of deaths[c]		Hospital beds[d]	
Private prepaid plans as % of private expenditure on health[a]	Per capita total expenditure on health at average exchange rate[a] (US$)	Per capita total expenditure on health at international dollar rate[a]	Per capita government expenditure on health at average exchange rate[a] (US$)	Per capita government expenditure on health at international dollar rate[a]				
2004	2004	2004	2004	2004	(%)	Year	per 10 000 population	Year
2.1	771	1 412	687	1 259	100	2004	84	2005
0.0	<1	47	<1	40	<25	2002	132	2002
...	5	15	1	4	<25	2002	...	
9.2	3 897	2 780	3 207	2 287	100	2001	38	2004
1.4	53	87	37	60	<25	2002	16	2000
...	215	309	153	221	>75	1999	39	2004
21.1	148	377	47	119	49	1999	22	2005
5.8	127	261	52	107	69	2003	14	2003
0.3	66	258	25	99	90	2001	22	2005
5.6	184	375	82	167	73	1999	9	2005
0.0	168	223	130	172	<25	2002	22	2005
0.0	10	27	4	11	<25	2002	...	
0.3	463	752	352	571	100	2003	58	2004
1.9	6	21	3	11	<25	2002	2	2004
...	148	284	92	177	100	2000	26	1999
10.3	2 664	2 203	2 057	1 700	100	2004	70	2005
57.3	3 464	3 040	2 715	2 382	100	2002	75	2004
...	231	264	159	182	<25	2002	...	
...	19	88	5	24	<25	2002	8	2005
1.8	60	171	16	47	64	2001	38	2005
39.1	3 521	3 171	2 709	2 440	100	2004	84	2005
6.6	27	95	12	40	<25	1999	9	2005
4.3	1 879	2 179	992	1 150	91	2003	47	2004
...	293	480	213	349	...		48	2005
4.2	127	256	52	105	86	1999	7	2005
0.0	22	96	3	13	<25	2002	...	
0.0	9	28	2	8	<25	2002	...	
...	56	329	47	275	...		29	2001
...	33	82	13	32	7	1999	8	2000
9.0	77	197	42	108	...		10	2002
3.2	800	1 308	573	937	100	2003	79	2005
0.0	4 413	3 294	3 679	2 746	96	2003	75	2002
0.8	31	91	5	16	<25	2000	7	2002
5.9	33	118	11	41	<25	2002	6	1998
4.4	158	604	75	288	38	2001	17	2005
...	58[h]	135[h]	45[h]	106[h]	<25	2002	13	2005
32.7	3 234	2 618	2 570	2 080	100	2002	57	2004
25.0	1 534	1 972	1 073	1 380	100	2003	63	2005
3.6	2 580	2 414	1 936	1 812	98	2001	40	2004
32.1	176	223	95	121	...		17	2005
1.9	2 823	2 293	2 295	1 864	100	2003	129	2001
7.4[i]	200[i]	502[i]	97[i]	243[i]	37	2004	17	2005
...	109	264	65	158	79	2003	78	2005
6.1	20	86	9	37	<10	1999	19	2002
0.0	112	271	104	252	>75	2002	15	2004

Health systems

Figures have been computed by WHO to ensure comparability; thus they are not necessarily the official statistics of Member States, which may use alternative rigorous methods.

	Member State	WHO region	Health expenditure ratios						
			Total expenditure on health as % of gross domestic product[a]	General government expenditure on health as % of total expenditure on health[a,b]	Private expenditure on health as % of total expenditure on health[a,b]	General government expenditure on health as % of total government expenditure[a]	External resources for health as % of total expenditure on health[a]	Social security expenditure on health as % of general government expenditure on health[a]	Out-of-pocket expenditure as % of private expenditure on health[a]
			2004	2004	2004	2004	2004	2004	2004
91	Kuwait	EMR	2.8	77.6	22.4	6.0	0.0	0.0	90.4
92	Kyrgyzstan	EUR	5.6	40.9	59.1	8.3	15.1	14.6	94.3
93	Lao People's Democratic Republic	WPR	3.9	20.5	79.5	5.0	10.2	12.1	90.3
94	Latvia	EUR	7.1	56.6	43.4	11.1	0.3	78.3	98.3
95	Lebanon	EMR	11.6	27.4	72.6	9.3	1.7	48.8	82.2
96	Lesotho	AFR	6.5	84.2	15.8	13.4	8.7	0.0	18.2
97	Liberia	AFR	5.6	63.9	36.1	20.1	37.8	0.0	98.5
98	Libyan Arab Jamahiriya	EMR	3.8	74.9	25.1	6.1	0.0	...	100.0
99	Lithuania	EUR	6.5	75.0	25.0	15.8	3.1	83.3	96.8
100	Luxembourg	EUR	8.0[j]	90.4[j]	9.6[j]	16.7[j]	0.0[j]	80.3[j]	69.9[j]
101	Madagascar	AFR	3.0	59.1	40.9	8.7	45.5	...	52.5
102	Malawi	AFR	12.9	74.7	25.3	28.8	59.4	0.0	35.2
103	Malaysia	WPR	3.8	58.8	41.2	7.5	0.1	0.7	74.1
104	Maldives	SEAR	7.7	81.4	18.6	16.0	1.6	29.2	100.0
105	Mali	AFR	6.6	49.2	50.8	12.8	13.8	...	99.5
106	Malta	EUR	9.2	76.1	23.9	14.4	0.0	0.0	90.2
107	Marshall Islands	WPR	15.2	97.0	3.0	14.5	16.9	15.7	100.0
108	Mauritania	AFR	2.9	69.4	30.6	5.3	20.2	0.0	100.0
109	Mauritius	AFR	4.3	54.7	45.3	9.8	1.4	...	80.8
110	Mexico	AMR	6.5	46.4	53.6	12.9	0.3	67.3	94.4
111	Micronesia (Federated States of)	WPR	7.6	85.7	14.3	10.2	71.9	...	40.0
112	Monaco	EUR	9.9	75.7	24.3	16.4	0.0	98.5	82.2
113	Mongolia	WPR	6.0	66.6	33.4	9.4	4.6	38.6	92.3
114	Montenegro	EUR	...	...	...	...	...	...	...
115	Morocco	EMR	5.1	34.3	65.7	5.5	0.9	0.0	76.0
116	Mozambique	AFR	4.0	68.4	31.6	9.1	55.9	0.0	38.5
117	Myanmar	SEAR	2.2	12.9	87.1	1.4	13.1	3.2	99.4
118	Namibia	AFR	6.8	69.0	31.0	13.5	16.9	1.7	18.1
119	Nauru	WPR	8.1	73.0	27.0	32.9	7.8	0.0	100.0
120	Nepal	SEAR	5.6	26.3	73.7	8.1	17.6	0.0	88.1
121	Netherlands	EUR	9.2	62.4	37.6	12.4	0.0	95.5	20.6
122	New Zealand	WPR	8.4	77.4	22.6	18.2	0.0	0.0	76.1
123	Nicaragua	AMR	8.2	47.1	52.9	12.0	11.3	26.3	95.9
124	Niger	AFR	4.2	52.5	47.5	10.3	21.3	...	85.1
125	Nigeria	AFR	4.6	30.4	69.6	3.5	5.6	0.0	90.4
126	Niue	WPR	15.1	98.8	1.2	12.4	43.2	0.0	100.0
127	Norway	EUR	9.7	83.5	16.5	17.8	0.0	16.3	95.2
128	Oman	EMR	3.0	81.4	18.6	6.1	0.0	0.0	57.1
129	Pakistan	EMR	2.2	19.6	80.4	1.9	2.5	0.0	98.0
130	Palau	WPR	9.7	91.2	8.8	16.4	19.8	0.0	100.0
131	Panama	AMR	7.7	66.9	33.1	10.4	0.2	49.9	82.5
132	Papua New Guinea	WPR	3.6	84.3	15.7	10.0	26.5	0.0	46.4
133	Paraguay	AMR	7.7	33.7	66.3	15.3	1.9	37.4	72.2
134	Peru	AMR	4.1	46.9	53.1	9.0	1.3	47.9	79.2
135	Philippines	WPR	3.4	39.8	60.2	6.3	3.6	23.8	77.9

Private prepaid plans as % of private expenditure on health[a]	Health expenditure aggregates				Coverage of vital registration of deaths[c]		Hospital beds[d]	
	Per capita total expenditure on health at average exchange rate[a] (US$)	Per capita total expenditure on health at international dollar rate[a]	Per capita government expenditure on health at average exchange rate[a] (US$)	Per capita government expenditure on health at international dollar rate[a]				
2004	2004	2004	2004	2004	(%)	Year	per 10 000 population	Year
9.6	633	538	491	417	90	2002	19	2005
...	24	102	10	42	71	2004	51	2005
0.5	17	74	3	15	<25	2002	9	2002
1.7	418	852	237	482	100	2004	77	2005
15.4	670	817	184	224	19	1999	36	2005
...	49	139	42	117	<25	2002	...	
0.0	9	22	6	14	<25	2002	...	
0.0	195	328	146	246	<25	2002	34	2004
0.5	424	843	318	633	100	2004	81	2005
17.6[j]	5 904[j]	5 178[j]	5 335[j]	4 679[j]	100	2004	63	2004
11.1	7	29	4	17	<25	2002	...	
14.6	19	58	14	43	<25	2002	...	
13.2	180	402	106	237	40	1998	18	2001
0.0	180	494	147	403	42	2003	23	2003
0.5	24	54	12	27	<25	2002	...	
7.3	1 239	1 733	943	1 318	100	2004	75	2005
0.0	272	555	264	539	53	1997	21	1999
0.0	15	43	10	30	<25	2002	6	2006
10.0	222	516	122	282	100	2003	30	2005
5.6	424	655	197	304	96	2002	10	2004
...	156	292	134	250	...		28	2000
17.8	5 330	4 744	4 037	3 593	...		...	
0.0	37	141	25	94	86	2003	75	2002
...	...	...	...	...	...		42	2005
24.0	82	234	28	80	34	1997	9	2004
0.6	12	42	8	29	<25	1997	...	
0.0	5[k]	38[k]	1[k]	5[k]	<25	2000	6	2000
77.2	190	407	131	281	<25	2002	...	
0.0	347	399	253	292	...		60	2004
0.0	14	71	4	19	<25	2002	2	2001
50.6	3 442	3 092	2 146	1 928	100	2004	50	2003
22.6	2 040	2 081	1 578	1 610	99	2000	60	2002
3.2	67	231	32	109	59	2002	9	2004
11.7	9	26	5	14	<25	2002	...	
6.7	23	53	7	16	<25	2002	12	2000
0.0	1 225	245	1 211	242	>75	2000	73	2003
0.0	5 405	4 080	4 512	3 406	96	2003	42	2005
28.6	295	419	240	341	71	2001	21	2005
...	14	48	3	9	<25	2002	7	2003
0.0	656	841	598	767	>75	1999	44	1998
17.5	343	632	229	423	89	2003	24	2004
6.2	30	147	26	124	...		...	
13.9	88	327	30	110	74	2000	12	2005
17.5	104	235	49	111	51	2000	11	2004
12.1	36	203	14	81	85	1998	12	2002

Health systems

Figures have been computed by WHO to ensure comparability; thus they are not necessarily the official statistics of Member States, which may use alternative rigorous methods.

	Member State	WHO region	Health expenditure ratios						
			Total expenditure on health as % of gross domestic product[a]	General government expenditure on health as % of total expenditure on health[a,b]	Private expenditure on health as % of total expenditure on health[a,b]	General government expenditure on health as % of total government expenditure[a]	External resources for health as % of total expenditure on health[a]	Social security expenditure on health as % of general government expenditure on health[a]	Out-of-pocket expenditure as % of private expenditure on health[a]
			2004	2004	2004	2004	2004	2004	2004
136	Poland	EUR	6.2	68.6	31.4	10.0	0.1	82.4	89.6
137	Portugal	EUR	9.8[j]	71.6[j]	28.4[j]	15.1[j]	0.0[j]	1.2[j]	79.4[j]
138	Qatar	EMR	2.4	76.5	23.5	6.1	0.0	0.0	86.4
139	Republic of Korea	WPR	5.5	52.6	47.4	10.3	0.0	79.2	80.4
140	Republic of Moldova	EUR	7.4	56.8	43.2	12.1	4.8	70.2	96.0
141	Romania	EUR	5.1	66.1	33.9	11.1	25.0	83.4	93.4
142	Russian Federation	EUR	6.0	61.3	38.7	9.8	0.1	36.2	76.7
143	Rwanda	AFR	7.5	56.8	43.2	16.5	37.1	4.6	36.9
144	Saint Kitts and Nevis	AMR	5.2	63.2	36.8	9.6	1.8	0.0	100.0
145	Saint Lucia	AMR	5.0	65.0	35.0	10.8	0.7	4.8	100.0
146	Saint Vincent and the Grenadines	AMR	6.1	63.2	36.8	11.0	0.1	0.0	100.0
147	Samoa	WPR	5.3	76.8	23.2	13.1	12.4	1.2	78.0
148	San Marino	EUR	7.4	79.0	21.0	21.6	0.0	94.0	96.8
149	Sao Tome and Principe	AFR	11.5	86.2	13.8	13.1	53.3	0.0	100.0
150	Saudi Arabia	EMR	3.9	76.5	23.5	9.9	0.0	...	26.4
151	Senegal	AFR	5.9	40.3	59.7	9.8	12.8	14.7	94.5
152	Serbia	EUR	...	...	...	...	...	...	...
153	Seychelles	AFR	6.1	75.3	24.7	10.2	2.4	3.3	62.5
154	Sierra Leone	AFR	3.3	59.0	41.0	7.8	35.4	0.0	100.0
155	Singapore	WPR	3.7	34.0	66.0	6.2	0.0	25.9	96.9
156	Slovakia	EUR	7.2	73.8	26.2	13.7	0.0	86.3	73.1
157	Slovenia	EUR	8.7	75.6	24.4	13.8	...	90.3	39.5
158	Solomon Islands	WPR	5.9	94.5	5.5	18.8	60.8	0.0	55.9
159	Somalia	EMR	...	...	...	...	...	...	...
160	South Africa	AFR	8.6	40.4	59.6	10.8	0.5	4.3	17.2
161	Spain	EUR	8.1	70.9	29.1	14.7	0.0	7.4	81.0
162	Sri Lanka	SEAR	4.3	45.6	54.4	8.4	1.2	0.2	84.0
163	Sudan	EMR	4.1	35.4	64.6	7.2	5.1	12.5	98.1
164	Suriname	AMR	7.8	46.0	54.0	9.7	9.7	36.7	60.2
165	Swaziland	AFR	6.3	63.8	36.2	11.2	9.5	0.0	40.2
166	Sweden	EUR	9.1	84.9	15.1	13.6	0.0	0.0	92.0
167	Switzerland	EUR	11.5	58.5	41.5	18.6	0.0	70.8	76.7
168	Syrian Arab Republic	EMR	4.7	47.4	52.6	5.9	0.2	0.0	100.0
169	Tajikistan	EUR	4.4	21.6	78.4	4.6	9.1	0.0	97.3
170	Thailand	SEAR	3.5	64.7	35.3	11.2	0.3	10.2	74.7
171	The former Yugoslav Republic of Macedonia	EUR	8.0	71.0	29.0	17.1	1.4	97.5	100.0
172	Timor-Leste	SEAR	11.2	78.9	21.1	15.0	53.7	0.0	25.6
173	Togo	AFR	5.5	20.7	79.3	6.9	8.9	14.4	84.9
174	Tonga	WPR	6.3	79.5	20.5	16.1	31.4	...	84.9
175	Trinidad and Tobago	AMR	3.5	38.9	61.1	5.1	0.2	0.0	88.5
176	Tunisia	EMR	6.2	52.1	47.9	8.8	0.2	19.4	83.0
177	Turkey	EUR	7.7	72.3	27.7	14.3	0.0	54.8	69.1
178	Turkmenistan	EUR	4.8	68.9	31.1	14.9	0.4	6.1	100.0
179	Tuvalu	WPR	16.6[m]	94.8[m]	5.2[m]	18.3[m]	46.5[m]	0.0[m]	16.5[m]
180	Uganda	AFR	7.6	32.7	67.3	10.0	25.2	0.0	51.3

	Health expenditure aggregates				Coverage of vital registration of deaths[c]		Hospital beds[d]	
Private prepaid plans as % of private expenditure on health[a]	Per capita total expenditure on health at average exchange rate[a] (US$)	Per capita total expenditure on health at international dollar rate[a]	Per capita government expenditure on health at average exchange rate[a] (US$)	Per capita government expenditure on health at international dollar rate[a]				
2004	2004	2004	2004	2004	(%)	Year	per 10 000 population	Year
1.9	411	814	282	559	100	2003	53	2004
15.9[j]	1 665[j]	1 897[j]	1 193[j]	1 359[j]	100	2003	37	2004
...	992	688	759	526	83	2001	24	2005
7.1	777	1 135	409	597	90	2002	66	2002
1.1	46	138	26	79	83	2004	64	2005
0	178	433	,17	286	100	2004	66	2005
9.9	245	583	150	358	97	2004	97	2005
1.3	16	126	9	72	<25	2002	17	2004
...	500	710	316	448	>75	1997	55	2005
...	232	302	151	196	100	2001	28	2005
...	210	418	133	264	99	1999	45	2004
0.0	109	218	84	167	28	2002	15	2002
3.2	3 356	3 198	2 652	2 527	>75	2000	...	
0.0	48	141	41	122	...		32	2003
43.7	412	601	315	460	31	2002	23	2004
4.4	39	72	16	29	<25	2002	...	
...	...	...	...	...	...		59	2005
0.0	534	634	403	478	>75	2000	...	
0.0	7	34	4	20	<25	2002	4	2006
...	943	1 118	321	381	82	2002	28	2003
0.0	565	1 061	417	782	100	2002	69	2005
51.7	1 438	1 815	1 087	1 372	100	2003	48	2005
0.0	35	114	33	108	28	1999	22	2003
...	...	...	...	...	<25	2002	...	
77.5	390	748	158	302	...		...	
16.2	1 971	2 099	1 397	1 488	100	2003	35	2003
8.8	43	163	19	74	...		30	2001
...	25	54	9	19	<25	2002	7	2004
0.8	194	376	89	173	...		31	2004
21.1	146	367	93	234	<25	2002	...	
1.9	3 532	2 828	3 000	2 402	100	2002	52	1997
21.1	5 572	4 011	3 261	2 347	100	2002	57	2004
0.0	58[l]	109[l]	27[l]	52[l]	100	2000	13	2004
0.0	14	54	3	12	50	2001	62	2005
16.5	88	293	57	190	91	2002	22	2000
...	212	471	150	335	90	2003	47	2005
0.0	44	143	34	113	<25	2002	...	
4.0	18	63	4	13	<10	2001	9	2005
0.4	117	316	93	251	<75	1998	29	2004
6.1	329	523	128	203	94	2000	33	2003
15.3	175	502	91	262	6	1999	18	2004
12.5	325	557	235	402	41	2003	26	2005
0.0	124	245	86	169	76	1998	49	2004
0.0[m]	355[m]	257[m]	337[m]	244[m]	>75	2000	40	2001
0.2	19	135	6	44	<25	2002	7	2004

Health systems

Figures have been computed by WHO to ensure comparability; thus they are not necessarily the official statistics of Member States, which may use alternative rigorous methods.

	Member State	WHO region	Health expenditure ratios						
			Total expenditure on health as % of gross domestic product[a]	General government expenditure on health as % of total expenditure on health[a,b]	Private expenditure on health as % of total expenditure on health[a,b]	General government expenditure on health as % of total government expenditure[a]	External resources for health as % of total expenditure on health[a]	Social security expenditure on health as % of general government expenditure on health[a]	Out-of-pocket expenditure as % of private expenditure on health[a]
			2004	2004	2004	2004	2004	2004	2004
181	Ukraine	EUR	6.5	56.7	43.3	9.4	0.7	0.0	90.5
182	United Arab Emirates	EMR	2.9	69.9	30.1	8.1	0.0	0.0	71.0
183	United Kingdom	EUR	8.1	86.3	13.7	15.9	0.0	0.0	91.8
184	United Republic of Tanzania	AFR	4.0	43.6	56.4	8.5	27.1	1.8	83.2
185	United States of America	AMR	15.4	44.7	55.3	18.9	0.0	28.0	23.8
186	Uruguay	AMR	8.2	43.5	56.5	10.1	0.3	42.0	31.1
187	Uzbekistan	EUR	5.1	46.6	53.4	7.8	3.9	...	96.2
188	Vanuatu	WPR	4.1	76.8	23.2	13.6	22.9	0.0	57.5
189	Venezuela (Bolivarian Republic of)	AMR	4.7	42.0	58.0	8.2	0.0	22.8	88.3
190	Viet Nam	WPR	5.5	27.1	72.9	5.0	2.0	16.9	88.0
191	Yemen	EMR	5.0	38.3	61.7	5.7	15.0	...	95.5
192	Zambia	AFR	6.3	54.7	45.3	12.8	36.3	0.0	71.4
193	Zimbabwe	AFR	7.5	46.1	53.9	8.9	13.1	0.0	48.7
194	The former state union of Serbia and Montenegro[e]	EUR	10.1[e]	72.1[e]	27.9[e]	14.0[e]	0.5[e]	81.7[e]	88.2[e]

Region								
African Region	AFR	6.0	43.9	56.1	8.8	9.2	6.3	49.2
Region of the Americas	AMR	12.7	47.5	52.5	17.4	0.1	25.1	32.4
South-East Asia Region	SEAR	4.0	27.3	72.7	4.5	2.2	7.3	89.5
European Region	EUR	8.6	74.2	25.8	14.3	0.1	49.9	70.1
Eastern Mediterranean Region	EMR	5.0	49.0	51.0	7.6	1.1	18.4	88.0
Western Pacific Region	WPR	5.8	56.9	43.1	13.1	0.3	61.6	85.6
Global		8.7	55.9	44.1	14.3	0.3	39.9	52.2

... Data not available or not applicable; AFR, African Region; AMR, Region of the Americas; SEAR, South-East Asia Region; EUR, European Region; EMR, Eastern Mediterranean Region; WPR, Western Pacific Region.

The global values for rates and ratios are weighted averages; for absolute numbers they are the sums of all WHO regions.

Expenditure estimates from the following countries should be interpreted with caution since they are derived from limited sources (mostly macro-economics data that are publicly accessible): Afghanistan, Angola, Comoros, Democratic People's Republic of Korea, Gabon, Guinea-Bissau, Iraq, Liberia, Libyan Arab Jamahiriya, Mauritania, Sierra Leone, Turkmenistan.

Expenditure estimates for countries that are members of the Organisation for Economic Co-operation and Development (OECD) are based on *OECD health data updates 2006* [online source]. Paris, OECD Publishing, 2006 (also available at http://www.oecd.org/health/healthdata) and subsequent updates from national correspondents.

New reports from national health accounts; surveys; updated national accounts series from sources such as the United Nations, the World Bank, the International Monetary Fund or other organizations; and other information or consultations with countries provided new bases for health expenditure estimates for the following countries: Bangladesh, Benin, Bhutan, Cambodia, China, Congo, Democratic Republic of the Congo, Equatorial Guinea, Ethiopia, Georgia, Ghana, India, Kyrgyzstan, Lao People's Democratic Republic, Malawi, Maldives, Mali, Mongolia, Nepal, Niger, Pakistan, Papua New Guinea, Philippines, Rwanda, Samoa, Sao Tome and Principe, Sri Lanka, Sudan, Thailand, Tonga, United Republic of Tanzania, Viet Nam and Zambia.

[a] National health accounts: country information. Geneva, World Health Organization, 2007 (http://www.who.int/nha/country).

[b] In some cases the sum of the ratios of general government expenditure and private expenditure on health may not add up to 100 because of rounding.

[c] WHO mortality database: tables. Geneva, World Health Organization, 2007 (http://who.int/healthinfo/morttables).

[d] Sources: *Health situation in the Americas: basic indicators 2006*. Washington, DC, Pan American Health Organization, 2006 (http://www.paho.org/english/dd/ais/BI-brochure-2006.pdf, accessed 1 March 2007); *Demographic and health indicators for countries of the Eastern Mediterranean: 2006*. Alexandria, World Health Organization Regional Office for the Eastern Mediterranean, 2006; *European health for all database (HFA-DB)*. Copenhagen, World Health Organization Regional Office for Europe, 2007 (http://data.euro.who.int/hfadb, accessed 1 March 2007); *Core indicators 2005*. New Delhi, WHO, Regional Office for South-East Asia, 2005 (http://www.searo.who.int/EN/Section1243/Section1382/Section1386_9855.htm, accessed 1 March 2007); *Core indicators 2005*. Manila, WHO, Regional Office for the Western Pacific, 2005 (http://www.wpro.who.int/information_sources/databases/core_indicators, accessed 1 March 2007); additional data compiled by WHO, Regional Office for Africa.

World Health Statistics 2007

	Health expenditure aggregates				Coverage of vital registration of deaths[e]		Hospital beds[d]	
Private prepaid plans as % of private expenditure on health[a]	Per capita total expenditure on health at average exchange rate[a] (US$)	Per capita total expenditure on health at international dollar rate[a]	Per capita government expenditure on health at average exchange rate[a] (US$)	Per capita government expenditure on health at international dollar rate[a]	(%)	Year	per 10 000 population	Year
2004	2004	2004	2004	2004				
1.2	90	427	51	242	99	2004	87	2005
18.4	711	503	497	352	65	2000	22	2002
8.2	2 900	2 560	2 502	2 209	100	2003	39	2004
4.8	12	29	5	12	<25	2002	...	
66.4	6 096	6 096	2 725	2 725	100	2002	33	2003
68.9	315	784	137	341	100	2000	24	2005
0.0	23	160	11	75	80	2002	52	2005
...	58	123	45	95	12	2000	20	2003
3.8	196	285	82	120	97	2002	9	2003
2.9	30	184	8	50	<25	2002	14	2002
...	34	82	13	31	<25	2002	6	2005
0.6	30	63	16	34	17	2000	20	2004
27.8	27	139	13	64	36	2001	...	
11.8[o]	219[o]	436[o]	158[o]	315[o]	90	2002	...	
40.6	48	108	22	47	...		...	
59.4	2 336	2 720	1 084	1 291	...		25	
2.5	31	99	8	27	...		9	
22.4	1 537	1 564	1 162	1 161	...		64	
7.8	91	224	50	110	...		13	
6.1	332	480	233	273	...		31	
39.7	645	777	382	434	...		26	

[e] Gross domestic product (GDP) includes income from both licit and illicit (opium) sources. Previous releases of World health statistics reported only licit GDP.
[f] Estimates do not include expenditures for the Hong Kong and Macao Special Administrative Regions.
[g] Benchmark revision of the gross domestic product lowers relative health expenditure compared with previous releases of World health statistics.
[h] Estimates do not include expenditures incurred in northern Iraq.
[i] Public expenditure on health includes contributions made by the United Nations Relief and Works Agency for Palestine Refugees in the Near East (UNRWA) to Palestinian refugees residing in Jordan.
[j] Changes in classifications linked to the health account systems led to changes as compared to previous releases.
[k] The market exchange rate was used this year instead of the official exchange rates, which were used in previous releases.
[l] The exchange rate used is the rate from the Central Bank of Syria for non-commercial transactions.
[m] Large amounts of funds from external sources, mainly for capital expenditures, resulted in high expenditures on health.
[n] See footnote o to the table on Health status: mortality.
[o] Estimates do not include expenditures incurred in the provinces of Kosovo and Metohia.

Inequities in health

Figures have been computed by WHO to ensure comparability; thus they are not necessarily the official statistics of Member States, which may use alternative rigorous methods.

	Member State	WHO region	Year	Probability of dying aged < 5 years per 1 000 live births[a] (under-5 mortality rate)									Children aged < 5 years stunted for age[a] (%)					
				Place of residence			Wealth quintile			Educational level of mother[a]			Place of residence			Wealth quintile		
				Rural	Urban	Ratio rural–urban	Lowest	Highest	Ratio lowest–highest	Lowest	Highest	Ratio lowest–highest	Rural	Urban	Ratio rural–urban	Lowest	Highest	Ratio lowest–highest
1	Armenia[c]	EUR	2000	59.2	37.3	1.6	60.9	29.6	2.1	89.1	48.1	1.9	16.0	10.1	1.6	19.0	9.3	2.0
2	Bangladesh	SEAR	2004	97.7	92.2	1.1	121.0	72.0	1.7	113.7	68.2	1.7	44.3	37.7	1.2	54.4	25.0	2.2
3	Benin	AFR	2001	175.5	133.6	1.3	198.2	93.1	2.1	174.5	80.8	2.2	33.4	24.2	1.4	35.4	18.2	1.9
4	Bolivia	AMR	2003	113.4	76.8	1.5	105.0	32.0	3.3	144.5	48.0	3.0	36.9	18.6	2.0	41.8	5.4	7.7
5	Botswana	AFR	1988	55.2	55.3	1.0	...	...	...	62.0	46.3	1.3	...	...	...	...	...	...
6	Brazil	AMR	1996	79.4	49.1	1.6	98.9	33.3	3.0	119.1	37.0	3.2	19.0	7.8	2.4	23.1	2.4	9.6
7	Burkina Faso	AFR	2003	201.5	136.4	1.5	206.0	144.0	1.4	198.4	108.0	1.8	41.4	19.8	2.1	45.7	20.6	2.2
8	Burundi	AFR	1987	184.2	163.7	1.1	...	...	...	191.2	80.7	2.4	48.6	27.1	1.8	...	...	...
9	Cambodia	WPR	2000	126.0	92.6	1.4	154.8	63.6	2.4	135.5	75.2	1.8	45.4	37.6	1.2	52.6	27.5	1.9
10	Cameroon	AFR	2004	168.8	119.3	1.4	189.0	88.0	2.1	185.7	93.3	2.0	38.2	23.1	1.7	40.9	12.3	3.3
11	Central African Republic[d]	AFR	1994–1995	178.4	128.6	1.4	192.9	98.3	2.0	175.2	83.1	2.1	37.2	28.6	1.3	42.3	25.0	1.7
12	Chad	AFR	2004	208.0	179.0	1.2	176.0	187.0	0.9	200.0	143.0	1.4	43.0	32.3	1.3	50.7	31.7	1.6
13	Colombia[e]	AMR	2005	33.0	23.0	1.4	39.0	16.0	2.4	51.0	16.0	3.2	17.1	9.5	1.8	19.8	3.3	6.0
14	Comoros[d]	AFR	1996	122.6	80.7	1.5	128.9	86.6	1.5	120.6	74.5	1.6	35.0	29.9	1.2	44.8	23.3	1.9
15	Côte d'Ivoire	AFR	1998–1999	196.8	125.2	1.6	...	...	...	192.7	79.4	2.4	28.6	18.3	1.6	...	...	...
16	Dominican Republic	AMR	2002	46.9	41.1	1.1	...	...	...	81.5	29.5	2.8	11.0	7.7	1.4	...	...	...
17	Ecuador	AMR	1987	112.2	65.0	1.7	...	...	...	158.9	49.0	3.2	...	...	...	...	...	...
18	Egypt	EMR	2005	56.1	39.1	1.4	74.6	25.1	3.0	67.7	30.7	2.2	18.4	16.2	1.1	23.6	14.4	1.6
19	El Salvador	AMR	1985	103.8	68.6	1.5	...	...	...	126.9	29.7	4.3	...	...	...	...	...	...
20	Eritrea	AFR	2002	117.1	86.1	1.4	100.0	65.0	1.5	120.6	58.5	2.1	42.6	27.8	1.5	44.8	17.6	2.5
21	Ethiopia	AFR	2005	135.0	98.0	1.4	130.0	92.0	1.4	139.0	54.0	2.6	47.9	29.8	1.6	47.9	34.9	1.4
22	Gabon	AFR	2000	99.9	88.4	1.1	93.1	55.4	1.7	112.0	87.1	1.3	29.0	17.4	1.7	32.8	11.5	2.9
23	Ghana	AFR	2003	118.3	92.7	1.3	128.0	88.0	1.5	124.9	84.5	1.5	34.0	19.9	1.7	41.8	13.2	3.2
24	Guatemala	AMR	1998–1999	68.5	57.8	1.2	77.6	39.3	2.0	78.5	42.3	1.9	54.4	32.4	1.7	65.3	7.5	8.7
25	Guinea	AFR	2005	204.0	133.0	1.5	217.0	113.0	1.9	194.0	92.0	2.1	38.4	22.6	1.7	41.3	21.8	1.9
26	Haiti	AMR	2000	149.4	111.7	1.3	163.9	108.7	1.5	150.5	74.0	2.0	26.5	11.5	2.3	30.8	7.4	4.2
27	India[d]	SEAR	1998–1999	111.4	65.4	1.7	141.3	45.5	3.1	124.4	50.5	2.5	48.5	35.7	1.4	58.1	26.7	2.2
28	Indonesia	SEAR	2002–2003	64.7	42.3	1.5	77.0	22.0	3.5	90.1	36.8	2.4	...	...	...	...	...	...
29	Jordan	EMR	2002	36.4	27.2	1.3	...	...	...	43.6	26.4	1.7	12.8	7.0	1.8	...	...	...
30	Kazakhstan[f]	EUR	1999	73.2	50.1	1.5	81.9	44.8	1.8	67.4	55.0	1.2	12.3	5.8	2.1	15.3	7.5	2.0
31	Kenya	AFR	2003	116.9	93.5	1.3	149.0	91.0	1.6	126.5	62.9	2.0	32.0	23.8	1.3	38.1	19.2	2.0
32	Kyrgyzstan[d,f]	EUR	1997	82.2	58.2	1.4	96.4	49.3	2.0	93.4	55.7	1.7	27.7	14.8	1.9	33.9	14.3	2.4
33	Liberia	AFR	1986	239.7	217.8	1.1	...	...	...	242.1	176.1	1.4	...	...	...	...	...	...
34	Madagascar	AFR	2003–2004	120.0	73.3	1.6	141.8	49.4	2.9	148.6	65.4	2.3	48.9	40.9	1.2	50.5	38.2	1.3
35	Malawi	AFR	2004	164.0	116.0	1.4	183.0	111.0	1.6	181.0	86.0	2.1	49.2	37.8	1.3	53.9	32.0	1.7
36	Mali	AFR	2001	253.2	184.6	1.4	247.8	148.1	1.7	246.9	89.6	2.8	42.1	23.2	1.8	44.8	19.7	2.3
37	Mauritania	AFR	2000–2001	96.2	110.7	0.9	98.1	78.5	1.2	110.5	85.5	1.3	37.9	30.2	1.3	38.7	23.4	1.7
38	Mexico	AMR	1987	104.2	49.7	2.1	...	...	...	114.1	28.8	4.0	...	...	...	...	...	...
39	Morocco	EMR	2003–2004	69.4	38.1	1.8	78.0	26.0	3.0	62.7	27.1	2.3	23.6	13.0	1.8	29.1	10.2	2.9
40	Mozambique	AFR	2003	192.0	143.2	1.3	196.0	108.0	1.8	200.5	85.7	2.3	45.7	28.5	1.6	49.3	20.0	2.5
41	Namibia	AFR	2000	66.1	49.5	1.3	55.4	31.4	1.8	83.6	47.1	1.8	23.0	21.7	1.1	26.7	15.3	1.7
42	Nepal	SEAR	2001	111.9	65.9	1.7	129.9	67.7	1.9	120.7	50.2	2.4	51.5	36.3	1.4	61.5	35.8	1.7
43	Nicaragua	AMR	2001	55.3	33.9	1.6	64.3	19.2	3.3	71.8	24.9	2.9	29.0	11.4	2.5	35.2	4.5	7.8
44	Niger[d]	AFR	1998	327.4	178.1	1.8	281.8	183.7	1.5	314.0	129.6	2.4	43.0	31.2	1.4	41.9	32.3	1.3
45	Nigeria	AFR	2003	242.7	152.9	1.6	257.0	79.0	3.3	269.4	107.2	2.5	42.9	28.9	1.5	48.8	17.9	2.7
46	Pakistan	EMR	1990–1991	131.9	93.6	1.4	124.5	73.8	1.7	128.4	64.7	2.0	54.5	40.4	1.3	61.1	32.9	1.9
47	Paraguay	AMR	1990	48.1	44.8	1.1	57.2	20.1	2.8	77.6	28.9	2.7	17.9	8.9	2.0	22.5	3.0	7.5
48	Peru	AMR	2000	85.3	39.0	2.2	92.6	17.6	5.3	106.0	35.1	3.0	40.2	13.4	3.0	47.0	4.5	10.4
49	Philippines	WPR	2003	52.2	30.4	1.7	66.0	21.0	3.1	104.7	28.5	3.7	...	...	...	...	...	...
50	Rwanda	AFR	2005	192.0	122.0	1.6	211.0	122.0	1.7	210.0	95.0	2.2	47.3	33.1	1.4	55.1	29.7	1.9

			Births attended by skilled health personnel[a] (%)									Measles immunization coverage among 1-year-olds[a] (%)								
Educational level of mother[b]			Place of residence			Wealth quintile			Educational level of mother[b]			Place of residence			Wealth quintile			Educational level of mother[b]		
Lowest	Highest	Ratio lowest–highest	Rural	Urban	Ratio urban–rural	Lowest	Highest	Ratio highest–lowest	Lowest	Highest	Ratio highest–lowest	Rural	Urban	Ratio urban–rural	Lowest	Highest	Ratio highest–lowest	Lowest	Highest	Ratio highest–lowest
21.0	13.0	1.6	94.5	99.1	1.0	93.3	100.0	1.1	89.9	96.8	1.1	72.1	76.0	1.1	67.8	74.1	1.1	90.8	74.3	0.8
50.4	31.6	1.6	9.1	29.6	3.3	3.4	39.6	11.6	4.3	28.0	6.5	73.9	82.8	1.1	59.5	90.5	1.5	62.3	87.7	1.4
33.0	17.1	1.9	68.4	82.9	1.2	49.6	99.3	2.0	67.6	98.6	1.5	64.1	75.3	1.2	56.9	83.1	1.5	63.4	88.6	1.4
44.4	12.7	3.5	38.6	77.7	2.0	34.4	98.9	2.9	29.8	90.0	3.0	60.2	66.5	1.1	62.3	73.7	1.2	60.6	74.0	1.2
...	...	...	71.7	93.5	1.3	...	...	...	53.6	96.6	1.8	69.9	65.4	0.9	...	...	...	67.8	63.0	0.9
21.2	5.9	3.6	73.3	92.3	1.3	71.6	98.6	1.4	66.0	94.5	1.4	76.5	90.2	1.2	77.9	90.2	1.2	67.4	90.6	1.3
40.8	12.4	3.3	30.5	87.7	2.9	38.8	90.8	2.3	32.7	94.7	2.9	53.3	73.1	1.4	48.3	71.3	1.5	54.3	80.4	1.5
49.0	24.6	2.0	16.8	85.2	5.1	...	...	...	15.6	75.7	4.9	47.8	51.1	1.1	...	...	...	45.2	56.3	1.2
51.1	34.9	1.5	28.0	57.2	2.0	14.7	81.2	5.5	19.3	65.8	3.4	54.6	61.0	1.1	43.9	81.8	1.9	45.6	71.1	1.6
40.1	21.0	1.9	44.2	84.2	1.9	29.3	94.5	3.2	22.9	91.7	4.0	58.3	72.5	1.2	52.1	83.2	1.6	46.1	79.3	1.7
37.2	24.1	1.5	23.7	77.7	3.3	14.3	81.7	5.7	29.4	84.8	2.9	40.5	68.4	1.7	31.3	79.8	2.5	38.6	79.2	2.1
44.3	22.1	2.0	6.4	45.6	7.1	3.6	55.4	15.4	9.3	66.7	7.2	19.2	37.5	2.0	8.2	38.1	4.6	18.2	53.7	3.0
27.3	3.5	7.8	91.1	98.9	1.1	89.2	99.7	1.1	84.1	100.0	1.2	75.8	85.1	1.1	69.4	90.0	1.3	70.0	92.6	1.3
38.2	25.0	1.5	43.1	78.9	1.8	26.2	84.8	3.2	40.8	82.9	2.0	63.5	63.0	1.0	51.1	86.0	1.7	58.7	75.5	1.3
28.3	14.2	2.0	32.1	79.1	2.5	...	...	...	37.9	83.6	2.2	58.8	82.0	1.4	...	...	...	57.8	94.6	1.6
12.8	5.5	2.3	95.7	99.0	1.0	...	...	...	89.4	99.4	1.1	86.0	89.5	1.0	...	...	...	70.1	93.0	1.3
...	...	...	39.0	84.5	2.2	...	...	...	31.3	88.2	2.8	...	...	...	...	...	...	...	...	...
21.5	14.8	1.5	65.8	88.7	1.3	50.5	95.7	1.9	54.3	89.1	1.6	96.5	96.8	1.0	95.1	97.2	1.0	96.0	97.6	1.0
...	...	...	79.1	93.3	1.2	...	...	...	73.3	99.0	1.4	76.9	85.2	1.1	...	...	...	66.3	88.0	1.3
44.6	16.2	2.8	10.4	64.7	6.2	6.7	81.0	12.1	12.0	87.9	7.3	78.5	93.8	1.2	83.8	96.4	1.2	77.1	95.6	1.2
49.1	24.0	2.0	2.6	44.6	17.2	0.7	26.6	38.0	2.3	57.7	25.1	32.2	65.4	2.0	24.9	52.5	2.1	30.0	63.4	2.1
22.5	16.5	1.4	69.4	92.9	1.3	67.2	97.1	1.4	83.9	92.9	1.1	37.1	61.1	1.6	34.1	71.3	2.1	42.3	63.9	1.5
38.0	23.7	1.6	30.9	79.7	2.6	20.6	90.4	4.4	29.7	67.9	2.3	81.8	85.8	1.0	75.0	88.8	1.2	78.2	89.3	1.1
64.4	12.7	5.1	25.0	66.1	2.6	8.8	91.9	10.4	21.8	84.8	3.9	83.4	86.0	1.0	79.5	91.1	1.1	72.9	95.4	1.3
35.9	18.9	1.9	25.6	80.7	3.2	14.5	87.4	6.0	32.8	84.1	2.6	48.9	54.8	1.1	42.0	57.2	1.4	47.7	67.6	1.4
27.9	9.7	2.9	11.0	52.2	4.7	4.1	70.0	17.1	10.0	62.0	6.2	50.2	60.9	1.2	42.9	63.3	1.5	43.8	69.9	1.6
54.9	30.6	1.8	33.5	73.3	2.2	16.4	84.4	5.1	23.6	74.0	3.1	45.3	69.2	1.5	28.4	81.2	2.9	34.0	75.8	2.2
...	...	...	55.2	78.9	1.4	...	...	...	32.4	85.6	2.6	66.2	77.6	1.2	...	...	...	41.9	83.2	2.0
20.4	7.5	2.7	96.8	98.8	1.0	...	...	...	90.7	98.7	1.1	94.2	95.4	1.0	...	...	...	80.8	95.9	1.2
12.3	6.8	1.8	99.5	98.4	1.0	99.2	98.5	1.0	99.7	98.3	1.0	76.2	81.4	1.1	73.8	75.7	1.0	86.7	89.4	1.0
36.4	19.0	1.9	34.5	72.0	2.1	17.0	75.4	4.4	15.8	72.0	4.6	69.7	85.9	1.2	54.8	88.0	1.6	51.1	84.9	1.7
32.4	18.6	1.7	97.8	99.2	1.0	96.0	100.0	1.0	97.7	99.0	1.0	84.5	83.7	1.0	81.9	80.7	1.0	85.1	77.5	0.9
...	...	...	44.9	76.7	1.7	...	...	...	49.3	86.6	1.8	28.0	30.2	1.1	...	...	...	24.9	42.7	1.7
49.1	38.0	1.3	39.6	70.6	1.8	29.9	93.9	3.1	21.9	80.5	3.7	55.9	73.9	1.3	38.4	84.0	2.2	36.1	85.2	2.4
52.4	33.1	1.6	53.0	83.8	1.6	46.6	84.6	1.8	42.8	83.4	1.9	77.6	86.8	1.1	67.4	88.3	1.3	72.1	93.9	1.3
40.1	13.6	2.9	26.6	80.8	3.0	8.1	81.9	10.1	34.4	90.8	2.6	41.3	70.8	1.7	39.7	76.5	1.9	44.9	78.7	1.8
37.1	21.4	1.7	28.9	85.8	3.0	14.7	92.8	6.3	40.4	91.6	2.3	53.0	74.3	1.4	42.0	86.2	2.1	55.4	79.8	1.4
...	...	...	44.0	85.9	2.0	...	...	...	29.7	95.4	3.2	52.6	62.3	1.2	...	...	...	45.7	64.1	1.4
21.8	10.4	2.1	39.5	85.3	2.2	29.5	95.4	3.2	48.8	94.4	1.9	85.9	94.2	1.1	83.1	97.6	1.2	87.6	96.3	1.1
47.7	14.5	3.3	34.1	80.7	2.4	24.8	88.6	3.6	31.4	94.8	3.0	70.8	90.8	1.3	60.8	96.4	1.6	65.6	99.1	1.5
28.5	17.9	1.6	66.3	93.1	1.4	55.4	97.1	1.8	46.8	89.1	1.9	78.4	84.3	1.1	76.2	85.7	1.1	69.5	83.3	1.2
54.9	32.8	1.7	10.2	51.1	5.0	3.6	45.1	12.5	6.6	45.9	7.0	69.9	80.6	1.2	61.1	83.2	1.4	63.2	92.9	1.5
35.7	8.7	4.1	83.1	96.5	1.2	77.5	99.3	1.3	76.9	97.8	1.3	74.1	77.1	1.0	76.2	93.8	1.2	69.4	72.8	1.0
42.3	23.6	1.8	8.1	68.7	8.5	4.2	62.8	15.0	13.8	68.5	5.0	27.8	67.1	2.4	23.0	65.8	2.9	31.8	73.9	2.3
50.5	20.0	2.5	27.1	58.8	2.2	13.0	84.5	6.5	13.8	75.0	5.4	28.5	52.1	1.8	15.9	70.7	4.4	15.6	66.5	4.3
55.0	23.8	2.3	8.1	42.4	5.2	4.6	55.2	12.0	11.0	62.3	5.7	43.6	64.6	1.5	27.9	74.8	2.7	43.6	76.5	1.8
21.5	5.8	3.7	48.3	87.0	1.8	41.2	98.1	2.4	32.3	93.5	2.9	52.4	65.0	1.2	48.0	68.7	1.4	31.8	71.1	2.2
51.6	12.6	4.1	25.3	84.6	3.3	13.0	87.5	6.7	14.7	84.5	5.7	82.2	86.1	1.0	80.8	92.3	1.1	75.8	88.4	1.2
...	...	...	40.8	79.0	1.9	25.1	92.4	3.7	11.0	71.8	6.5	77.5	81.8	1.1	69.7	89.4	1.3	45.6	83.3	1.8
50.3	43.3	1.2	34.6	63.1	1.8	27.2	66.4	2.4	27.2	72.9	2.7	85.0	89.6	1.1	84.9	87.6	1.0	82.6	92.0	1.1

Inequities in health

Figures have been computed by WHO to ensure comparability; thus they are not necessarily the official statistics of Member States, which may use alternative rigorous methods.

	Member State	WHO region	Year	Probability of dying aged < 5 years per 1 000 live births[a] (under-5 mortality rate)									Children aged < 5 years stunted for age[a] (%)					
				Place of residence			Wealth quintile			Educational level of mother[b]			Place of residence			Wealth quintile		
				Rural	Urban	Ratio rural–urban	Lowest	Highest	Ratio lowest–highest	Lowest	Highest	Ratio lowest–highest	Rural	Urban	Ratio rural–urban	Lowest	Highest	Ratio lowest–highest
51	Senegal	AFR	1999	171.2	92.1	1.9	...	...	...	159.9	80.1	2.0	...	...	...	...	...	...
52	South Africa	AFR	1998	71.2	43.2	1.6	87.4	21.9	4.0	83.8	45.6	1.8	...	...	...	...	...	...
53	Sri Lanka	SEAR	1987	42.8	39.9	1.1	...	...	...	71.7	36.2	2.0	28.6	19.3	1.5	...	...	...
54	Sudan	EMR	1990	144.0	117.0	1.2	...	...	...	151.9	84.3	1.8	...	...	...	...	...	...
55	Thailand	SEAR	1987	51.7	34.3	1.5	...	...	...	75.9	20.6	3.7	24.2	11.2	2.2	...	...	...
56	Togo[d]	AFR	1998	157.4	101.3	1.6	167.7	97.0	1.7	159.1	82.5	1.9	23.9	14.8	1.6	29.0	11.0	2.6
57	Trinidad and Tobago	AMR	1987	30.4	38.7	0.8	...	...	...	69.0	40.1	1.7	4.6	5.0	0.9	...	...	...
58	Tunisia	EMR	1988	85.3	62.1	1.4	...	...	...	84.1	38.9	2.2	24.5	11.8	2.1	...	...	...
59	Turkey	EUR	1998	73.5	51.3	1.4	85.0	32.6	2.6	84.0	31.7	2.6	22.0	12.6	1.7	28.5	3.7	7.7
60	Turkmenistan	EUR	2000	99.8	72.7	1.4	105.5	69.8	1.5	133.3	88.3	1.5	24.1	19.5	1.2	25.1	17.1	1.5
61	Uganda	AFR	2000–2001	163.8	100.5	1.6	191.8	106.4	1.8	186.9	93.0	2.0	39.9	26.5	1.5	43.3	25.1	1.7
62	United Republic of Tanzania	AFR	2004–2005	138.0	108.0	1.3	137.0	93.0	1.5	160.0	76.0	2.1	40.5	25.8	1.6	44.9	15.7	2.9
63	Uzbekistan[c]	EUR	2002	87.5	53.4	1.6	...	...	...	102.2	35.5	2.9	23.8	16.3	1.5	...	...	...
64	Viet Nam[d]	WPR	2002	35.6	16.2	2.2	...	...	...	66.2	28.6	2.3	...	...	...	...	...	...
65	Yemen	EMR	1997	128.2	95.8	1.3	163.1	73.0	2.2	126.1	70.6	1.8	55.7	40.3	1.4	57.7	34.9	1.7
66	Zambia	AFR	2001–2002	182.3	140.0	1.3	191.7	92.4	2.1	197.8	121.1	1.6	51.1	37.1	1.4	54.1	31.6	1.7
67	Zimbabwe	AFR	1999	99.7	69.0	1.4	99.5	62.2	1.6	118.8	78.7	1.5	29.2	20.6	1.4	32.7	18.6	1.8

...Data not available or not applicable; AFR, African Region; AMR, Region of the Americas; SEAR, South-East Asia Region; EUR, European Region; EMR, Eastern Mediterranean Region; WPR, Western Pacific Region.

[a] Sources: Figures stratified by "place of residence" and "educational level of mother" were extracted from Demographic and Health Survey data using STATcompiler software (http://www.measuredhs.com/). For surveys conducted in 2001 or earlier, figures stratified by "wealth quintile" were extracted from Gwatkin et al. *Initial country-level differences about socio-economic differences in health, nutrition and population.* 2nd ed. Washington, DC, World Bank, 2003; for surveys conducted after 2001, the figures were extracted from Demographic and Health Survey reports.

[b] Lowest educational level achieved by mother is "no education"; highest level is "secondary or higher".

[c] Lowest educational level achieved by mother is "primary".

WORLD HEALTH STATISTICS 2007

	Births attended by skilled health personnel[a] (%)										Measles immunization coverage among 1-year-olds[a] (%)									
Educational level of mother[b]			Place of residence			Wealth quintile			Educational level of mother[b]			Place of residence			Wealth quintile			Educational level of mother[b]		
Lowest	Highest	Ratio lowest–highest	Rural	Urban	Ratio urban–rural	Lowest	Highest	Ratio highest–lowest	Lowest	Highest	Ratio highest–lowest	Rural	Urban	Ratio urban–rural	Lowest	Highest	Ratio highest–lowest	Lowest	Highest	Ratio highest–lowest
...	...	...	75.7	95.6	1.3	...	...	...	78.5	97.1	1.2	58.1	78.7	1.4	...	...	...	54.0	90.9	1.7
...	...	...	75.5	93.4	1.2	67.8	98.1	1.4	59.7	91.4	1.5	79.3	85.1	1.1	73.5	84.5	1.1	64.0	85.6	1.3
50.0	21.0	2.4	86.0	94.8	1.1	...	...	...	67.7	92.2	1.4	67.1	62.8	0.9	...	...	...	47.0	73.5	1.6
...	...	...	59.3	85.9	1.4	...	...	...	52.6	95.5	1.8	56.3	69.9	1.2	...	...	...	50.3	84.8	1.7
30.5	9.4	3.2	59.9	95.6	1.6	...	...	...	43.7	95.9	2.2	15.7	35.2	2.2	...	...	...	11.2	37.5	3.3
25.5	12.0	2.1	39.8	86.4	2.2	25.1	91.2	3.6	36.7	86.8	2.4	38.2	58.0	1.5	34.5	63.2	1.8	36.5	63.7	1.7
16.7	4.0	4.2	97.2	98.3	1.0	...	...	...	91.7	98.1	1.1	30.5	35.9	1.2	...	...	...	60.0	37.2	0.6
22.4	4.9	4.6	50.2	87.4	1.7	...	...	...	54.2	97.1	1.8	77.1	91.0	1.2	...	...	...	77.0	93.9	1.2
33.4	5.4	6.2	68.7	87.7	1.3	53.4	98.2	1.8	51.1	97.6	1.9	72.7	82.2	1.1	63.9	88.9	1.4	57.0	89.7	1.6
25.7	22.3	1.2	96.6	98.2	1.0	96.8	98.3	1.0	92.7	97.3	1.0	92.0	81.8	0.9	92.1	91.8	1.0	74.1	87.6	1.2
45.5	28.9	1.6	33.1	80.4	2.4	19.7	77.3	3.9	21.5	75.8	3.5	55.3	68.4	1.2	49.1	64.5	1.3	54.1	69.4	1.3
41.2	19.1	2.2	47.4	83.3	1.8	38.6	89.5	2.3	39.9	88.6	2.2	77.7	89.7	1.2	65.2	90.9	1.4	64.6	89.8	1.4
19.5	19.2	1.0	...	...	...	...	...	...	...	...	...	...	...	...	...	...	...	...	...	...
...	...	...	82.2	99.0	1.2	58.1	99.7	1.7	41.6	93.7	2.3	80.7	94.3	1.2	64.4	97.8	1.5	49.2	93.1	1.9
54.4	29.4	1.9	14.3	46.9	3.3	6.8	49.7	7.3	16.4	62.5	3.8	33.8	71.9	2.1	15.7	72.9	4.6	37.2	74.2	2.0
53.8	36.1	1.5	27.6	79.0	2.9	19.7	91.1	4.6	17.3	77.8	4.5	83.9	85.5	1.0	81.2	88.4	1.1	79.8	87.2	1.1
35.3	22.5	1.6	64.2	89.4	1.4	56.7	93.5	1.6	42.8	85.6	2.0	75.7	86.2	1.1	80.2	85.8	1.1	69.4	85.2	1.2

[d] Data for "Children aged < 5 years stunted for age" and "Births attended by skilled health personnel" correspond to births occurring in the 3 years preceding the survey not 5 years.
[e] Highest educational level achieved by mother is "higher than secondary".
[f] Lowest educational level achieved by mother is "primary or secondary"; highest level is "higher than secondary-special".
[g] Lowest educational level achieved by mother is "primary or middle school"; highest level is "higher than secondary-special".

Demographic and socioeconomic statistics

Figures have been computed by WHO to ensure comparability; thus they are not necessarily the official statistics of Member States, which may use alternative rigorous methods.

	Member State	WHO region	Population			Total fertility rate[a]	Adolescent fertility rate[c]	
			No.[a]	Annual growth rate[a]	In urban areas[b]			
			('000s) 2005	(%) 1995–2005	(%) 2005	(per woman) 2005	(%)	Year
1	Afghanistan	EMR	29 863	3.7	23	7.3	9.3	1999
2	Albania	EUR	3 130	0.0	45	2.2	1.5	2004
3	Algeria	AFR	32 854	1.5	63	2.4	2.7	1999
4	Andorra	EUR	67	0.4	91	1.2	0.6	2004
5	Angola	AFR	15 941	2.6	53	6.6	...	
6	Antigua and Barbuda	AMR	81	1.6	39	2.2	...	
7	Argentina	AMR	38 747	1.1	90	2.3	6.2	2001
8	Armenia	EUR	3 016	−0.7	64	1.3	3.0	2004
9	Australia	WPR	20 155	1.2	88	1.7	1.6	2003
10	Austria	EUR	8 189	0.2	66	1.4	1.4	2004
11	Azerbaijan	EUR	8 411	0.8	52	1.8	3.1	2004
12	Bahamas	AMR	323	1.5	90	2.2	5.0	2000
13	Bahrain	EMR	727	2.2	97	2.4	1.4	2000
14	Bangladesh	SEAR	141 822	2.0	25	3.1	13.5	2003
15	Barbados	AMR	270	0.3	53	1.5	...	
16	Belarus	EUR	9 755	−0.5	72	1.2	2.2	2004
17	Belgium	EUR	10 419	0.3	97	1.7	1.0	1999
18	Belize	AMR	270	2.3	48	3.0	8.0	1998
19	Benin	AFR	8 439	3.1	40	5.6	13.3	1999
20	Bhutan	SEAR	2 163	2.2	11	4.1	8.2	1999
21	Bolivia	AMR	9 182	2.1	64	3.7	...	
22	Bosnia and Herzegovina	EUR	3 907	1.3	46	1.3	3.9	1999
23	Botswana	AFR	1 765	0.9	57	3.0	6.8	1999
24	Brazil	AMR	186 405	1.5	84	2.3	6.2	1998
25	Brunei Darussalam	WPR	374	2.4	74	2.4	3.1	2000
26	Bulgaria	EUR	7 726	−0.7	70	1.2	4.0	2002
27	Burkina Faso	AFR	13 228	3.0	18	6.5	13.1	2001
28	Burundi	AFR	7 548	2.1	10	6.8	6.2	1999
29	Cambodia	WPR	14 071	2.2	20	3.9	2.2	1999
30	Cameroon	AFR	16 322	2.1	55	4.4	14.1	2002
31	Canada	AMR	32 268	1.0	80	1.5	1.4	2003
32	Cape Verde	AFR	507	2.4	57	3.6	10.1	1999
33	Central African Republic	AFR	4 038	1.7	38	4.8	14.9	1999
34	Chad	AFR	9 749	3.3	25	6.7	19.3	2002
35	Chile	AMR	16 295	1.2	88	2.0	4.9	2003
36	China	WPR	1 323 345	0.8	40	1.7	0.3	2002
37	Colombia	AMR	45 600	1.7	73	2.5	9.2	2003
38	Comoros	AFR	798	2.8	37	4.6	7.0	1999
39	Congo	AFR	3 999	3.2	60	6.3	11.0	1999
40	Cook Islands	WPR	18	−1.1	70	2.6	5.0	2000
41	Costa Rica	AMR	4 327	2.2	62	2.2	7.7	2003
42	Côte d'Ivoire	AFR	18 154	2.1	45	4.8	...	
43	Croatia	EUR	4 551	−0.3	56	1.3	1.4	2004
44	Cuba	AMR	11 269	0.4	76	1.6	4.9	2003
45	Cyprus	EUR	835	1.3	69	1.6	0.6	2004
46	Czech Republic	EUR	10 220	−0.1	74	1.2	1.1	2004
47	Democratic People's Republic of Korea	SEAR	22 488	0.7	62	2.0	...	
48	Democratic Republic of the Congo	AFR	57 549	2.5	32	6.7	11.9	
49	Denmark	EUR	5 431	0.4	86	1.8	0.6	2004
50	Djibouti	EMR	793	2.7	86	4.8	19.0	1999
51	Dominica	AMR	79	0.5	73	1.9	...	
52	Dominican Republic	AMR	8 895	1.5	67	2.6	11.8	2001
53	Ecuador	AMR	13 228	1.5	63	2.7	5.6	1998
54	Egypt	EMR	74 033	1.9	43	3.1	4.8	2003
55	El Salvador	AMR	6 881	2.0	60	2.8	7.5	2003

Adult literacy rate[d]	Net primary school enrolment ratio[d]		Gross national income per capita[n]	Population living below the poverty line[f]	
(%) 2000–2004	Males (%)	Females (%)	(PPP int.$) 2005	% living on <US$1 per day	Year
	1999–2005				
28.1	...	...	...	...	
98.7	94	94	5 420	<2.0	2002
69.9	98	95	6 770	...	
...	90	87	...	...	
67.4	...	...	2 210	...	
...	...	...	11 700	...	
97.2	99	98	13 920	7.0	2003
99.4	92	95	5 060	<2.0	2003
...	96	96	30 610	...	
...	...	...	33 140	...	
98.8	85	83	4 890	<2.0	2002
...	88	90	...	...	
86.5	96	97	21 290	...	
42.6	92	95	2 090	36.0	2000
...	98	97	...	...	
99.6	91	88	7 890	<2.0	2002
...	99	99	32 640	...	
...	95	96	6 740	...	
34.7	93	72	1 110	30.9	2003
...	...	...	...	...	
86.7	95	96	2 740	23.2	2002
96.7	...	...	7 790	...	
81.2	81	83	10 250	...	
88.6	...	...	8 230	7.5	2003
92.7	...	...	...	...	
98.2	96	95	8 630	<2.0	2003
21.8	46	35	1 220	27.2	2003
59.3	60	54	640	54.6	1998
73.6	100	96	2 490	...	
67.9	...	...	2 150	17.1	2001
...	99	100	32 220	...	
78.0	92	91	6 000	...	
48.6	...	...	1 140	...	
25.7	68	46	1 470	...	
95.7	...	...	11 470	<2.0	2000
90.9	...	...	6 600	16.6	2001
92.8	83	84	7 420	7.0	2003
...	60	50	2 000	...	
...	...	...	810	...	
...	78	77	...	...	
94.9	...	...	9 680	2.2	2001
48.7	62	50	1 490	14.8	2002
98.1	88	87	12 750	<2.0	2001
99.8	97	95	...	...	
96.8	96	96	22 230	...	
...	...	...	20 140	...	
...	...	...	...	...	
67.2	...	...	720	...	
...	97	99	33 570	...	
...	36	28	2 240	...	
...	87	88	5 560	...	
87.0	85	87	7 150	2.5	2003
91.0	97	98	4 070	15.8	1998
71.4	97	94	4 440	3.1	1999–2000
81.1	92	92	5 120	19.0	2002

Demographic and socioeconomic statistics

Figures have been computed by WHO to ensure comparability; thus they are not necessarily the official statistics of Member States, which may use alternative rigorous methods.

	Member State	WHO region	Population			Total fertility rate[a]	Adolescent fertility rate[c]	
			No.[a]	Annual growth rate[a]	In urban areas[b]			
			('000s) 2005	(%) 1995–2005	(%) 2005	(per woman) 2005	(%)	Year
56	Equatorial Guinea	AFR	504	2.4	39	5.9	15.2	1999
57	Eritrea	AFR	4 401	3.6	19	5.3	8.5	2000
58	Estonia	EUR	1 330	–0.8	69	1.4	2.1	2003
59	Ethiopia	AFR	77 431	2.6	16	5.7	11.7	1999
60	Fiji	WPR	848	1.0	51	2.8	3.5	2002
61	Finland	EUR	5 249	0.3	61	1.7	1.1	2004
62	France	EUR	60 496	0.4	77	1.9	0.8	2003
63	Gabon	AFR	1 384	2.1	84	3.8	14.6	1999
64	Gambia	AFR	1 517	3.1	54	4.5	17.6	1999
65	Georgia	EUR	4 474	–1.2	52	1.4	4.7	2004
66	Germany	EUR	82 689	0.1	75	1.3	1.1	2004
67	Ghana	AFR	22 113	2.2	48	4.1	7.4	2001
68	Greece	EUR	11 120	0.4	59	1.2	1.1	2003
69	Grenada	AMR	103	0.3	31	2.3	5.3	2000
70	Guatemala	AMR	12 599	2.4	47	4.4	12.0	2000
71	Guinea	AFR	9 402	2.3	33	5.7	15.3	2003
72	Guinea-Bissau	AFR	1 586	2.9	30	7.1	9.1	1999
73	Guyana	AMR	751	0.3	28	2.2	...	
74	Haiti	AMR	8 528	1.4	39	3.8	8.0	1998
75	Honduras	AMR	7 205	2.5	46	3.5	13.7	1999
76	Hungary	EUR	10 098	–0.2	66	1.3	2.1	2004
77	Iceland	EUR	295	1.0	93	1.9	1.6	2003
78	India	SEAR	1 103 371	1.7	29	2.9	5.1	2000
79	Indonesia	SEAR	222 781	1.3	48	2.3	5.4	2001
80	Iran (Islamic Republic of)	EMR	69 515	1.1	67	2.1	3.5	2000
81	Iraq	EMR	28 807	2.9	67	4.5	1.7	2000
82	Ireland	EUR	4 148	1.4	60	2.0	1.9	2003
83	Israel	EUR	6 725	2.3	92	2.8	1.5	2004
84	Italy	EUR	58 093	0.1	68	1.3	0.7	2003
85	Jamaica	AMR	2 651	0.7	53	2.4	6.3	2004
86	Japan	WPR	128 085	0.2	66	1.3	0.6	2004
87	Jordan	EMR	5 703	2.9	82	3.3	3.0	2000
88	Kazakhstan	EUR	14 825	–0.7	57	1.9	2.6	2003
89	Kenya	AFR	34 256	2.3	21	5.0	11.6	2001
90	Kiribati	WPR	99	2.1	47	4.0	...	
91	Kuwait	EMR	2 687	4.7	98	2.3	1.5	2004
92	Kyrgyzstan	EUR	5 264	1.4	36	2.6	2.7	2004
93	Lao People's Democratic Republic	WPR	5 924	2.4	21	4.6	...	
94	Latvia	EUR	2 307	–0.8	68	1.3	1.6	2004
95	Lebanon	EMR	3 577	1.2	87	2.2	1.6	1999
96	Lesotho	AFR	1 795	0.6	19	3.4	9.8	2003
97	Liberia	AFR	3 283	4.4	58	6.8	18.0	1999
98	Libyan Arab Jamahiriya	EMR	5 853	2.0	85	2.9	1.4	2000
99	Lithuania	EUR	3 431	–0.6	67	1.3	1.9	2004
100	Luxembourg	EUR	465	1.4	83	1.7	1.1	2004
101	Madagascar	AFR	18 606	2.9	27	5.1	15.4	2001
102	Malawi	AFR	12 884	2.5	17	5.9	16.0	2003
103	Malaysia	WPR	25 347	2.2	67	2.8	1.2	2000
104	Maldives	SEAR	329	2.7	30	4.0	3.1	2000
105	Mali	AFR	13 518	2.9	30	6.8	19.2	1999
106	Malta	EUR	402	0.6	95	1.5	1.7	2002
107	Marshall Islands	WPR	62	2.0	67	4.3	...	
108	Mauritania	AFR	3 069	2.9	40	5.6	8.8	2001
109	Mauritius	AFR	1 245	1.0	42	2.0	3.7	2002
110	Mexico	AMR	107 029	1.5	76	2.3	9.4	2000

World Health Statistics 2007

Adult literacy rate[d]	Net primary school enrolment ratio[d]		Gross national income per capita[e]	Population living below the poverty line[f]	
(%) 2000–2004	Males (%)	Females (%)	(PPP int.$) 2005	% living on <US$1 per day	Year
	1999–2005				
87.0	92	78	7 580	...	
...	50	42	1 010	...	
99.8	94	94	15 420	<2.0	2003
45.2	58	55	1 000	23.0	1999–2000
...	97	96	5 960	...	
...	99	99	31 170	...	
...	99	99	30 540	...	
...	77	77	5 890	...	
...	73	77	1 920	59.3	1998
...	93	92	3 270	6.5	2003
...	...	...	29 210	...	
57.9	65	65	2 370	44.8	1998–1999
96.0	100	99	23 620	...	
...	84	84	7 260	...	
69.1	95	91	4 410	13.5	2002
29.5	69	58	2 240	...	
...	53	37	700	...	
...	94	92	4 230	...	
...	...	...	1 840	53.9	2001
80.0	90	92	2 900	20.7	1999
...	90	88	16 940	<2.0	2002
...	100	97	34 760	...	
61.0	92	87	3 460	34.7	1999–2000
90.4	95	93	3 720	7.5	2002
77.0	89	88	8 050	<2.0	1998
74.1	94	81	...	...	
...	96	96	34 720	...	
97.1	97	98	25 280	...	
98.4	99	99	28 840	...	
79.9	90	91	4 110	<2.0	2000
...	100	100	31 410	...	
89.9	90	92	5 280	<2.0	2002–2003
99.5	93	92	7 730	<2.0	2003
73.6	76	77	1 170	...	
...	96	98	...	...	
93.3	85	87	24 010	...	
98.7	90	90	1 870	<2.0	2003
68.7	87	82	2 020	27.0	2002
99.7	...	...	13 480	<2.0	2003
...	94	93	5 740	...	
82.2	83	88	3 410	...	
...	74	58	...	...	
...	...	...	...	...	
99.6	90	89	14 220	<2.0	2003
...	91	91	65 340	...	
70.7	89	89	880	61.0	2001
64.1	93	98	650	...	
88.7	93	93	10 320	...	
96.3	89	90	...	...	
19.0	50	43	1 000	...	
87.9	94	94	18 960	...	
...	90	89	...	...	
51.2	75	74	2 150	25.9	2000
84.4	94	95	12 450	...	
91.0	98	98	10 030	4.5	2002

Demographic and socioeconomic statistics

Figures have been computed by WHO to ensure comparability; thus they are not necessarily the official statistics of Member States, which may use alternative rigorous methods.

	Member State	WHO region	Population No.[a] ('000s) 2005	Population Annual growth rate[a] (%) 1995–2005	Population In urban areas[b] (%) 2005	Total fertility rate[a] (per woman) 2005	Adolescent fertility rate[c] (%)	Adolescent fertility rate[c] Year
111	Micronesia (Federated States of)	WPR	110	0.3	22	4.3	...	
112	Monaco	EUR	35	1.1	100	1.8	...	
113	Mongolia	WPR	2 646	1.0	57	2.3	2.8	2000
114	Montenegro	EUR	608	–0.2	...	1.8	...	
115	Morocco	EMR	31 478	1.5	59	2.7	3.5	2002
116	Mozambique	AFR	19 792	2.2	35	5.3	18.5	2001
117	Myanmar	SEAR	50 519	1.3	31	2.2	2.9	1999
118	Namibia	AFR	2 031	2.1	35	3.7	9.8	1999
119	Nauru	WPR	14	2.4	100	3.8	6.2	2000
120	Nepal	SEAR	27 133	2.3	16	3.5	11.6	2000
121	Netherlands	EUR	16 299	0.5	80	1.7	0.7	2003
122	New Zealand	WPR	4 028	1.0	86	2.0	2.7	2004
123	Nicaragua	AMR	5 487	2.1	59	3.1	9.8	2000
124	Niger	AFR	13 957	3.5	17	7.7	20.7	1999
125	Nigeria	AFR	131 530	2.4	48	5.6	12.6	2002
126	Niue	WPR	1	–2.1	37	2.8	...	
127	Norway	EUR	4 620	0.6	77	1.8	0.8	2004
128	Oman	EMR	2 567	1.7	71	3.4	3.6	1999
129	Pakistan	EMR	157 935	2.3	35	4.0	5.4	1999
130	Palau	WPR	20	1.4	70	1.8	...	
131	Panama	AMR	3 232	1.9	71	2.6	8.4	2002
132	Papua New Guinea	WPR	5 887	2.3	13	3.8	6.7	2000
133	Paraguay	AMR	6 158	2.5	58	3.7	6.5	2003
134	Peru	AMR	27 968	1.6	73	2.7	5.9	2002
135	Philippines	WPR	83 054	2.0	63	3.0	5.5	2001
136	Poland	EUR	38 530	0.0	62	1.2	1.4	2004
137	Portugal	EUR	10 495	0.5	58	1.5	1.9	2004
138	Qatar	EMR	813	4.5	95	2.9	1.9	2004
139	Republic of Korea	WPR	47 817	0.6	81	1.2	0.2	2004
140	Republic of Moldova	EUR	4 206	–0.3	47	1.2	2.9	2003
141	Romania	EUR	21 711	–0.4	54	1.3	3.3	2003
142	Russian Federation	EUR	143 202	–0.3	73	1.4	2.8	2004
143	Rwanda	AFR	9 038	5.2	19	5.5	3.6	1999
144	Saint Kitts and Nevis	AMR	43	0.6	32	2.3	6.4	2000
145	Saint Lucia	AMR	161	0.8	28	2.2	6.6	2001
146	Saint Vincent and the Grenadines	AMR	119	0.5	46	2.2	7.1	2000
147	Samoa	WPR	185	1.0	22	4.2	2.5	2000
148	San Marino	EUR	28	0.9	97	1.3	0.6	2003
149	Sao Tome and Principe	AFR	157	2.1	58	3.8	...	
150	Saudi Arabia	EMR	24 573	2.8	81	3.8	1.5	2004
151	Senegal	AFR	11 658	2.5	42	4.8	10.3	2002
152	Serbia	EUR	9 863	–0.3	...	1.8	...	
153	Seychelles	AFR	81	0.7	53	2.1	1.7	1999
154	Sierra Leone	AFR	5 525	2.9	41	6.5	16.2	1999
155	Singapore	WPR	4 326	2.2	100	1.3	0.7	2004
156	Slovakia	EUR	5 401	0.1	56	1.2	2.1	2002
157	Slovenia	EUR	1 967	0.0	51	1.2	0.6	2003
158	Solomon Islands	WPR	478	2.8	17	4.1	7.5	2000
159	Somalia	EMR	8 228	2.7	35	6.2	5.5	1999
160	South Africa	AFR	47 432	1.2	59	2.7	6.5	2001
161	Spain	EUR	43 064	0.8	77	1.3	1.0	2002
162	Sri Lanka	SEAR	20 743	0.9	15	1.9	1.5	1999
163	Sudan	EMR	36 233	2.1	41	4.2	9.2	1999
164	Suriname	AMR	449	0.8	74	2.5	6.2	2003
165	Swaziland	AFR	1 032	0.8	24	3.7	6.3	1999

Adult literacy rate[d]	Net primary school enrolment ratio[d]		Gross national income per capita[a]	Population living below the poverty line[f]	
(%) 2000–2004	Males (%)	Females (%)	(PPP int.$) 2005	% living on <US$1 per day	Year
	1999–2005				
...	...	...	...	...	
	...	...		...	
97.8	84	84	2 190	27.0	1998
	...	...		...	
52.3	89	83	4 360	<2.0	1999
	75	67	1 270		
89.9	89	91	...	...	
85.0	71	76	7 910	...	
...	...	...	...	...	
48.6	83	73	1 530	24.1	2003–2004
...	99	98	32 480	...	
...	99	99	23 030	...	
76.7	89	87	3 650	45.1	2001
28.7	46	32	800	...	
	64	57	1 040	70.8	2003
...	99	98	...	...	
...	99	99	40 420	...	
81.4	77	79	14 680		
49.9	76	56	2 350	17.0	2002
...	98	94	...	...	
91.9	98	98	7 310	6.5	2002
57.3	...	...	2 370	...	
	...	...	4 970	16.4	2002
87.7	97	97	5 830	12.5	2002
92.6	93	95	5 300	15.5	2000
...	97	98	13 490	<2.0	2002
...	99	98	19 730	...	
89.0	95	94	...	...	
...	100	99	21 850	<2.0	1998
98.4	86	86	2 150	22.0	2001
97.3	92	92	8 940	<2.0	2003
99.4	91	92	10 640	<2.0	2002
64.9	72	75	1 320	51.7	1999–2000
...	91	98	12 500	...	
...	99	96	5 980	...	
...	95	92	6 460	...	
98.8	90	91	6 480	...	
...	...	...	...	...	
...	98	98	...	...	
79.4	62	56	14 740	...	
39.3	68	64	1 770	...	
...	...	...	...	...	
91.8	96	97	15 940	...	
35.1	...	...	780	...	
92.5	...	...	29 780	...	
...	...	...	15 760	...	
99.7	98	98	22 160	<2.0	1998
...	65	62	1 880	...	
...	...	...	...	...	
82.4	88	89	12 120	10.7	2000
...	100	99	25 820	...	
90.7	99	98	4 520	5.6	2002
60.9	47	39	2 000	...	
89.6	90	96	...	...	
79.6	76	77	5 190	...	

Demographic and socioeconomic statistics

Figures have been computed by WHO to ensure comparability; thus they are not necessarily the official statistics of Member States, which may use alternative rigorous methods.

	Member State	WHO region	Population			Total fertility rate[a]	Adolescent fertility rate[c]	
			No.[a]	Annual growth rate[a]	In urban areas[b]			
			('000s) 2005	(%) 1995–2005	(%) 2005	(per woman) 2005	(%)	Year
166	Sweden	EUR	9 041	0.2	84	1.7	0.7	2002
167	Switzerland	EUR	7 252	0.4	75	1.4	0.5	2002
168	Syrian Arab Republic	EMR	19 043	2.6	51	3.3	6.0	1999
169	Tajikistan	EUR	6 507	1.2	25	3.6	5.6	1999
170	Thailand	SEAR	64 233	1.0	32	1.9	3.5	2000
171	The former Yugoslav Republic of Macedonia	EUR	2 034	0.4	69	1.5	2.3	2004
172	Timor-Leste	SEAR	947	1.1	26	7.8	...	
173	Togo	AFR	6 145	3.1	40	5.1	9.1	1999
174	Tonga	WPR	102	0.5	24	3.3	...	
175	Trinidad and Tobago	AMR	1 305	0.4	12	1.6	...	
176	Tunisia	EMR	10 102	1.2	65	1.9	1.3	1999
177	Turkey	EUR	73 193	1.6	67	2.4	5.6	2000
178	Turkmenistan	EUR	4 833	1.4	46	2.6	2.3	1999
179	Tuvalu	WPR	10	0.6	48	3.6	...	
180	Uganda	AFR	28 816	3.3	13	7.1	20.7	1999
181	Ukraine	EUR	46 481	−1.0	68	1.1	2.9	2003
182	United Arab Emirates	EMR	4 496	6.3	77	2.4	4.4	1999
183	United Kingdom	EUR	59 668	0.3	90	1.7	2.7	2002
184	United Republic of Tanzania	AFR	38 329	2.2	24	4.8	13.9	2003
185	United States of America	AMR	298 213	1.0	81	2.0	4.3	2002
186	Uruguay	AMR	3 463	0.7	92	2.3	6.4	2002
187	Uzbekistan	EUR	26 593	1.5	37	2.6	4.0	2001
188	Vanuatu	WPR	211	2.1	23	3.9	4.2	2000
189	Venezuela (Bolivarian Republic of)	AMR	26 749	1.9	93	2.6	8.1	2002
190	Viet Nam	WPR	84 238	1.4	26	2.2	2.5	2000
191	Yemen	EMR	20 975	3.3	27	5.9	7.7	1999
192	Zambia	AFR	11 668	2.0	35	5.4	16.1	2000
193	Zimbabwe	AFR	13 010	1.0	36	3.4	1.1	1999
194	The former state union of Serbia and Montenegro[d]	EUR	...	...	52	...	2.4	2003

	Region							
	African Region	AFR	738 083	2.4	36	5.2	11.9	
	Region of the Americas	AMR	886 334	1.3	79	2.3	6.5	
	South-East Asia Region	SEAR	1 656 529	1.6	31	2.8	5.9	
	European Region	EUR	893 200	0.2	69	1.6	2.5	
	Eastern Mediterranean Region	EMR	538 001	2.2	48	3.7	4.9	
	Western Pacific Region	WPR	1 751 457	0.9	45	1.8	0.8	
	Global		6 463 605	1.3	49	2.6	5.0	

... Data not available or not applicable; AFR, African Region; AMR, Region of the Americas; SEAR, South-East Asia Region; EUR, European Region; EMR, Eastern Mediterranean Region; WPR, Western Pacific Region.

The global values for rates and ratios are weighted averages; for absolute numbers they are the sums of all WHO regions.

[a] *World population prospects: the 2004 revision* [CD-ROM extended data set]. New York, Population Division, Department of Economic and Social Affairs, United Nations Secretariat, 2005 (No. E.05.XIII.12).

[b] *World urbanization prospects: the 2005 revision* [CD-ROM edition] New York, United Nations, Department of Economic and Social Affairs, Population Division, 2006 (POP/DB/WUP/Rev.2005).

[c] *World fertility data 2006* [wall chart], New York, Population Division, Department of Economic and Social Affairs, United Nations Secretariat, 2006 (POP/DB/Fert/Rev.2006).

Adult literacy rate[d]	Net primary school enrolment ratio[d]		Gross national income per capita[e]	Population living below the poverty line[f]	
(%) 2000–2004	Males (%)	Females (%)	(PPP int.$) 2005	% living on <US$1 per day	Year
	1999–2005				
...	99	98	31 420	...	
...	94	94	37 080	...	
79.6	97	92	3 740	...	
99.5	99	94	1 260	7.4	2003
92.6	...	...	8 440	<2.0	2002
96.1	92	92	7 080	<2.0	2003
...	...	...	...	...	
53.2	85	72	1 550	...	
98.9	92	89	8 040	...	
98.8	92	92	13 170	...	
74.3	97	98	7 900	<2.0	2000
87.4	92	87	8 420	3.4	2003
98.8	...	...	...	...	
...	...	...	...	...	
66.8	...	...	1 500	...	
99.4	82	82	6 720	<2.0	2003
...	72	70	24 090	...	
...	99	99	32 690	...	
69.4	92	91	730	57.8	2000–2001
...	94	90	41 950	...	
98.0	...	...	9 810	<2.0	2003
...	...	...	2 020	...	
74.0	95	93	3 170	...	
93.0	92	92	6 440	8.3	2000
90.3	97	91	3 010	...	
53.0	87	63	920	15.7	1998
68.0	80	80	950	75.8	2002–2003
...	81	82	1 940	...	
96.4	96	96	...	...	

...	75	72	2 231	...	
...	...	...	20 611	...	
...	93	89	3 557	...	
...	95	94	18 887	...	
...	84	75	4 956	...	
...	...	...	8 951	...	
82.2	...	...	9 420	...	

[d] UNESCO Institute for Statistics Database. *Database access* [online database]. Montreal, UNESCO Institute for Statistics, 2007 (http://stats.uis.unesco.org, accessed 1 March 2007).

[e] PPP int.$, purchasing power parity at international dollar rate. Source: *GNI per capita 2005, atlas method and PPP.* Quick reference tables. Washington, DC, World Bank, 2006 (http://siteresources.worldbank.org/DATASTATISTICS/Resources/GNIPC.pdf, accessed 1 March 2007).

[f] World development indicators 2006. Washington, DC, International Bank for Reconstruction and Development, World Bank, 2006 (http://devdata.worldbank.org/wdi2006).

[g] See footnote o to the table on Health status: mortality.

www.ingramcontent.com/pod-product-compliance
Ingram Content Group UK Ltd.
Pitfield, Milton Keynes, MK11 3LW, UK
UKHW051523180426
11947UKWH00018B/1549

9 789241 563406